Holistic Thought in
Social Science

D. C. PHILLIPS

Holistic Thought in Social Science

STANFORD UNIVERSITY PRESS
Stanford, California

Stanford University Press
Stanford, California
© 1976 by the Board of Trustees of the
Leland Stanford Junior University
Printed in the United States of America
Cloth ISBN 0-8047-0923-8
Paper ISBN 0-8047-1015-5
Original edition 1976
Last figure below indicates year of this printing:
88 87 86 85 84 83 82 81 80 79

Acknowledgments

I WISH TO express my debt to Mrs. Barbara Falk and the late Dr. Elizabeth Gasking, of the University of Melbourne, who first fostered my critical interest in holism; to Professor P. W. Musgrave of Monash University in Melbourne, who commented on a number of draft chapters; to Professor J. W. N. Watkins, of the London School of Economics, to whose seminar I presented the substance of several chapters; and to colleagues and students at both Monash and Stanford universities. Cheerful secretarial assistance was given by Elaine Scott of Monash University and Dorothy Farana of Stanford, and the Index was prepared by Joanne Kliejunas.

Several chapters of the book incorporate material previously published in the *Journal of the History of Ideas* (1970), *Abacus* (1969), and the *Academy of Management Journal* (1972); this material is used with the kind consent of the editors.   D.C.P.

Contents

Holistic Thought in
Social Science

You may ... find much of the thinking of an individual, a school, or even a generation, dominated and determined by one or another turn of reasoning, trick of logic, methodological assumption, which if explicit would amount to a large and important and perhaps highly debatable proposition in logic or metaphysics.

Arthur O. Lovejoy

Introduction

IN ANCIENT ROME, legend has it, a plebeian revolt was once quelled when the tribune Menenius Agrippa argued to the mob that the state, like a living body, is a whole; and just as the parts of the body are interrelated and require each other's presence, so with the various strata of society. This organic analogy, and the associated concept of wholeness, seemed to gather strength with the centuries. They came into prominence in the modern world in the wake of the Romantic movement, were strengthened by their transformation into a logical principle in the philosophy of the Hegelians, and persisted to play an important role in twentieth-century biology, psychology, sociology, anthropology, historiography, and political and administrative theory. In fact, it has often been argued that holism is as important in these "human" sciences as the so-called mechanistic or analytic method is in the physical sciences.

There is an enormous body of literature on holism, but a student of any one of the fields of study just mentioned is unlikely to encounter it in any ordered way.

He is almost certain to meet at least a few holistic theses, and probably some of the arguments against them; but he is likely to remain ignorant of the full scope of holism. He may not realize that debates over methodological individualism or the place of psychological explanations in sociology are related to those over system theory, over organicism in biology and psychology, over structuralism and functionalism, and over internal relations in philosophy. And he can easily become confused: the difficulty of finding a clear statement of the central ideas of holism in the literature is notorious, and there is a corresponding difficulty in evaluating them.

Several important threads run through modern holistic writing, but they are seldom teased apart for the reader. In the first place, it is common to find holists attacking what they call the mechanistic or atomistic method; but although this "simple-minded epistemology of Galileo" is frequently rejected on the grounds that it is inadequate for dealing with complex wholes, the analyses of it that are presented to justify the rejection could themselves fairly be regarded as simple-minded.

Another thread linking many forms of contemporary holism is a strong opposition to reductionism—to explaining the characteristics of any complex entity in terms of the properties of its parts plus relevant covering laws. Interesting points have been made both in the attacks on reductionism and in its defense; but again, not all holists have taken sufficient care in mounting their arguments, and there are major confusions.

[2]

Introduction

As well as attacking the same targets, holists tend to affirm the same theses: "A part cannot be understood in isolation from the whole." "The parts of an organic whole are dynamically interrelated or interdependent." These and several other widely advanced claims can all be shown to be based on Hegel's principle of internal relations—in Arthur O. Lovejoy's words, a "large and important and perhaps highly debatable proposition in logic or metaphysics." Several neo-Hegelian philosophers of the late nineteenth century expounded the doctrine of internal relations in words that are closely mirrored by social and biological scientists of the twentieth century.

It is apparent, then, that holism is not a simple position, and it will not be portrayed as such. It will be argued in the following pages that holism is a complex of three major and separable theses, one of which can itself be analyzed as five interrelated ideas. The structure of the book cannot avoid reflecting something of this complexity, and the argument will not always develop along one clear line. The first three chapters, however, are closely interrelated, and it is here—in the context of philosophical and biological examples—that many of the key conceptual distinctions are introduced. Subsequent chapters, discussing material from the social sciences, will draw heavily on the ideas developed earlier.

This book was written in the belief that it is possible to discuss the relevant issues of holism clearly and in a way that will be of interest to the social scientist. But it does not attempt the impossible; and it does not purport to be a detailed treatise on Hegelian philosophy, modern system theory, or the nature of sociological theory. It is hoped, however, that the Bibliography (pp. 135–44) will guide the further reading of those who wish to pursue in greater depth the matters that are taken up.

I

Wholes and the Hegelians

O NE OF THE perennial problems in man's intellectual history has been finding the most appropriate
way to study any complex entity or system. Over the
centuries, many theorists have advocated what has been
loosely called the mechanistic or analytic method. Suppose that a clocklike object is presented for investigation.
The child, the adult, or even the scientist will inspect
the object, shake it, peer inside it, and perhaps dismantle
it. The components will be examined separately, and two
or more may be fitted together and examined as an as-
sembly. In this way the process of studying the parts and
gradually piecing them together will proceed. It is obvious that this is a piecemeal approach; it is analytic in
the sense that the entity of interest is divided into simple
component parts, which are investigated separately. To
take a more sophisticated example, the scientific study
of the behavior of gases first established a relationship
between only two of the many characteristics a gas possesses (pressure and volume, in Boyle's law). Then a

third factor was added (temperature, in Charles' law), and by degrees a complex picture was built up.

This piecemeal method of investigation, which will usually be called the analytic method in this book, has had its critics. It is not that the method is a poor one; rather, it has been argued that an analytic approach is simply not appropriate in dealing with an important class of entities. For example, if a living organism is under examination, studying its parts in isolation will produce artifacts, for when they are isolated they are no longer parts of a living system. How, then, is an organic whole to be approached?

It must have appeared to many men of the nineteenth century that this problem had been solved in the form of a set of five interrelated ideas pertaining to organic wholes; for purposes of identification this set of holistic theses will be called organicism, or *Holism 1*:

1. *The analytic approach as typified by the physico-chemical sciences proves inadequate when applied to certain cases—for example, to a biological organism, to society, or even to reality as a whole.*

2. *The whole is more than the sum of its parts.*

3. *The whole determines the nature of its parts.*

4. *The parts cannot be understood if considered in isolation from the whole.*

5. *The parts are dynamically interrelated or interdependent.*

All five ideas require clarification. Idea 1, that the analytic approach as typified by the physicochemical sciences is inadequate when applied to a biological organism or to reality as a whole, is perhaps the most important organismic idea; for the core of the organicists' position has been that the method of analysis typically practiced in the physicochemical sciences does not do justice to the type of relationship existing between the parts within an organic system. The parts of an organic system are internally related to each other, and when the nature of this internal relationship is spelled out in detail it produces the remaining four constituent ideas of organicism.

The theory of internal relations was popularized in the English-speaking world during the last half of the nineteenth century by an upsurge of interest in Hegelian philosophy that was largely inspired by opposition to the growing mechanism and materialism of science. At first the works of Hegel himself (1770–1831) and of commentators on Hegel were the chief influences; but later in the century there also appeared many neo-idealists whose thought diverged somewhat from Hegel's. Among the most interesting of these later writers were F. H. Bradley, A. E. Taylor, and J. McTaggart, and it is their expositions of internal relations that will be examined here.*

The points concerning internal relations that Bradley made in his *Appearance and Reality* (1893) will be taken

* By treating these three men together, and by including them under the convenient blanket term "organicists," it is not intended to imply that their views were identical. In fact, Taylor's view (1903) was close to that of Bradley (1893); but McTaggart's view (1921) was different in many respects. However, for the present purpose—discussion of the essential features of the theory of internal relations—it is the points of agreement rather than the differences that are important.

as the starting point. Consider the entities A, B, and C:

First, any relation between these entities is possible only within some "whole" that embraces them. Or as Bradley put it, "Everywhere there must be a whole embracing what is related, or there would be no differences and no relation."[1]

Second, entities are *altered* by the relationships into which they enter. A, B, and C would be different when isolated, compared with their condition when interrelated.[2]

Finally, the entities A, B, and C "qualify" the whole of which they are parts, and the whole in turn "qualifies" A, B, and C. "There is no identity or likeness possible except in a whole, and every such whole must qualify and be qualified by its terms. And, where the whole is different, the terms that qualify it and contribute to it must so far be different, and so far therefore by becoming elements in a fresh unity the terms must be altered."[3]

Bradley's second point is of vital importance. In effect, he maintained that when entity A enters into a relationship with entity B or C, it gains some property or characteristic, p, as a result of this relationship. Without the relationship, and hence without property p, Bradley argues, A would be different, or not-A. Any relation at all between A and another entity necessarily determines some property of A, without which A would not be what it is. This is the heart of the theory of internal relations: entities are *necessarily* altered by the relations into which they enter. On the other hand, to mechanists (or rather, analysts), relations do not alter the entities that are related. As Hegel remarked, "and this constitutes the characteristic of Mechanism, which is, that whatever relation relates the terms is foreign to them and does not concern their nature; even if it involves the appearance of a One, it remains nothing else than a collocation, mixture, heap, or the like."[4]

Bradley's argument has force as long as discussion centers around the "nature" of an entity; but much of this force is lost if the theory of internal relations is expressed in the philosophical terminology that has become commonplace since the middle of the twentieth century. Emphasis on the nature of entities has been replaced by emphasis on the defining and accompanying characteristics affecting the usage of terms. From this later point of view, Bradley appears to have been maintaining that as a result of its relationship with entity B or C, entity A would have some characteristic p, and that this characteristic would be one of the defining characteristics of A. Without A's relationship to B or C, the defining characteristic p would not exist, and A would in fact be not-A. Every relationship into which A entered, no matter what sort of relationship it was, would thus determine a defining characteristic of A. As McTaggart expressed the point, "If any part of the nature of A goes, the nature of A as a whole goes.... No quality of a substance, therefore, could be different while leaving the other unchanged."[5] This key organicist argument has been revived in recent years by the system theorists, as later chapters will demonstrate.

When phrased in terms of defining characteristics,

the theory of internal relations can be seen to face serious difficulties. The main problem is that not all the characteristics of an entity are defining characteristics, as many introductory philosophy texts are at pains to point out. Numerous characteristics are accompanying characteristics—they may always be present, but their presence or absence may not influence the identity or characterization of the entity. Thus even if it is admitted that every relation into which *A* enters determines some characteristic of *A*, it is not necessarily true that a characteristic so determined will be a defining characteristic of *A*. The characteristics determined by *some* relations will be defining, but those determined by others may not be.[6] It is possible, therefore, for *A* to enter into a relationship, yet remain unchanged; in this case the new characteristic that *A* acquires as a result of the relationship would be an accompanying and not a defining characteristic.[7]

Organicists cannot meet this difficulty by arguing that in using terminology everyone is free to stipulate which characteristics are to be taken as defining and which are only accompanying, and by charging that their opponents are capitalizing on this freedom and have arbitrarily reclassified some defining characteristics as accompanying. Despite some sound points, this argument fails to answer the central assertion: that all the features of an entity, including its multitudinous relational characteristics, cannot be taken as defining.

The influential philosophy of Ludwig Wittgenstein reinforces the attack on organicism here. In *Philosophical Investigations*, he pointed out that in many cases our usage of a term is not determined by the presence of a single defining characteristic, or even by a constant set of such characteristics. Rather, there is a cluster, or "family," of characteristics, and we may decide to apply a term even if only some of these are present.[8] This explains why we can use a single term ("democracy" is a good example) to cover cases with few features in common: different characteristics from the cluster are present in the various cases, but enough are present in each case to warrant use of the "family" name. Obviously, organicists hold the contrary view that if even one feature of entity A changes or is not present, this is enough to warrant its being called not-A.

A related difficulty with the theory of internal relations is that it renders the attainment of knowledge impossible. To have knowledge of A, in the sense of knowing the defining features of A, we must know all of A's relationships, since each of these determines a defining feature; but since A is related to everything else in the "whole" of which it is a part, this "whole" must be known completely before A can be known. This seems a difficult principle to put into practice. As Bertrand Russell remarked of Hegel, for whom the whole was the universe, "If all knowledge were knowledge of the universe as a whole, there would be no knowledge."[9]

The organicists' attitude toward the analytic method, which found expression in the first of the five theses making up Holism 1, was not motivated solely by their acceptance of the theory of internal (or organic) relations. In general, organicists misunderstood the analytic method itself, and especially the conditions necessary for the scientific analysis of any complex system, organic or inorganic. They did not realize that the law or laws applicable to that system had first to be known, and that the initial conditions of the system then had to be described.[10] For instance, to understand the behavior of a given mass of gas, physicists must know both the relevant gas laws (e.g. Boyle's law) and the values of such parameters as pressure, volume, and temperature at a particular instant of time. In rejecting the analytic method as inadequate, organicists overlooked the fact that their opponents had the difficult task of stating the initial conditions for extremely complex systems. And certainly, organicists advanced no argument to show that the laws and initial conditions of any complex system could not eventually be discovered; hence there is no reason to believe that analytically derived explanations of organic wholes will not be arrived at in the end.

The remaining four ideas constituting organicism are all closely linked to internal relations. Consider the second idea: the whole is more than the sum of its parts. The point the organicists were making here can again be explained in terms of the entities A, B, and C. The characteristics of the whole formed by these interrelated entities are *not* exactly the same as the totality of the separate characteristics of A, B, and C; rather, characteristics of the whole are more than the sum of the characteristics of the parts. According to the theory of internal relations, when the entities A, B, and C become interrelated they obtain new characteristics (call these X, Y, Z). Since

these characteristics do not exist in the isolated entities
A, B, and *C,* the simple total of characteristics when they
are in the unrelated state will not include the relational
characteristics *X, Y, Z.*

Organicists, however, would be likely to point out that
it is impossible to have unrelated entities; and they would
deny any possibility of dealing with *A, B,* or *C* in isolation. Entities are *always* interrelated, and always parts of
a whole. Therefore, the whole cannot be treated as a mere
grouping of its parts. In other words, the extra defining
qualities *X, Y, Z* are never really absent.

Several issues raised by this second idea of organicism
should be clarified. In the first place, the position outlined is not incompatible with the analytic method, for
analysts as well as organicists have recognized the importance of relations. An electronics engineer, for example, in studying a complex piece of equipment, does
not simply study each of its components in isolation; he
also studies the circuit, that is, the network of relationships between components. Furthermore, an electronic
circuit in fact contains elements whose properties are
modified by their interrelationships.

Second, organicists sometimes slide from arguing that
the whole is more than the sum of its parts into arguing
that *knowledge* of the whole cannot be obtained from
knowledge of the parts. This position is unwarranted,
because there are some wholes about which knowledge
can be obtained through the analytic method. As the
philosopher of science Ernest Nagel has written: "The
mere fact that we can now explain some features of

relatively highly organized bodies on the basis of theories formulated in terms of relations between relatively more simply structured elements—for example, the specific heats of solids in terms of quantum theory or the changes in phase of compounds in terms of thermodynamics of mixtures—should give us pause."[11]

However, it must be acknowledged that in some cases the analytic method appears to run into serious difficulty. Such cases usually involve the phenomenon of emergence. For example: A molecule of the compound water contains two parts of hydrogen and one part of oxygen in combination, hence the formula H_2O. If the hydrogen and oxygen atoms were studied in isolation, and their properties determined, it could not be deduced from this information that when combined they would form the colorless, odorless, and tasteless liquid we call "water." The combination of the atoms produces a substance with *emergent properties*. This is a case, organicists argue, where the whole is clearly more than the sum of the parts—where the properties of the whole (the emergent water molecule) can only be discovered by studying the whole.

The point overlooked in this argument is that organicists are in no more favorable a position to deal with emergence than analysts. Emergence has often been misconstrued because of failure to recognize a central point. As Nagel put it: "The logical point constituting the core of the doctrine of emergence is applicable to all areas of inquiry and is as relevant to the analysis of explanations within mechanics and physics generally as it is to discussions of the laws of other sciences."[12] The "logical point" here is that the conclusion of a valid deduction cannot contain an expression that does not appear in the premises; this is indeed the core of the issue, since both scientific explanations and scientific predictions can be put in the form of deductions. It follows that the existence of an emergent property cannot be deduced from premises that do not contain reference to this property. It is logically impossible, for example, to deduce (or predict) the production of a colorless, odorless, and tasteless liquid (i.e. water) from premises that refer only to the properties of the gaseous elements hydrogen and oxygen. But if the analytic method cannot deal satisfactorily with emergent properties, no other method can do any better, for the stumbling block is simply a lack of necessary information. (The theme of emergence has other aspects as well, as will appear in later sections.)

Another point arising from the second basic idea of organicism—"the whole is more than the sum of the parts"—is that the very term "sum" is far from clear. The rules by which the sum of a group of entities is determined will differ according to the type of entities under consideration. In mathematics and physics, for example, it is common to distinguish between arithmetic sum, algebraic sum, and vector sum. Moreover, it is quite possible to define a "sum" in such a way that the whole *is* more than the sum of its parts. But since organicists have not made a practice of stating explicitly just what they mean by this term, their claim embodied in Idea 2 is at best vague.

The third constituent idea of organicism, that the whole *determines* the nature of the parts, is even more paradoxical. As G. E. Moore commented in 1903, "That this supposition is self-contradictory a very little reflection should be sufficient to show."[13] In effect, the "supposition" suggests that the whole causes itself—the parts are embodied in the whole, and in determining the nature of these parts the whole is determining its own nature.

Once again the organicists' case was based on the theory of internal relations. If entities A, B, and C form a whole, then they must be interrelated. It then follows from the theory of internal relations that the natures (i.e. the defining characteristics) of these three entities will be determined at least in part by the relational properties they thus possess. If the whole were different from what it is—if, for example, entity D were part of it—then A, B, and C would be different from what they are. They would be related to the new entity D; hence each of them would have a new relational quality and, according to the theory of internal relations, a different nature. In other words, if the whole were different the parts would be different, and it is in this sense that the whole determines the nature of its parts. Or as McTaggart put it: "Now the essential feature of an organic entity is that the parts manifest the whole—that, since the whole as a unity is what it is, the parts must be what they are. This, as we have seen, is really the case with all wholes, and therefore all wholes are really organic unities."[14]

The fourth major idea in organicism was that the parts cannot be *understood* if considered in isolation from the whole. The term "understood" is an obvious source of vagueness, but the intention of organicists probably was to state that the nature of the parts (i.e. their defining characteristics) cannot be known if the parts are considered in isolation from the whole. This, at least, was the view expressed by A. E. Taylor: "No lesser system within the whole is entirely explicable in terms of its own internal structure. For a full understanding of the nature of the lesser system, and of the way in which it manifests a common character through the variety of its elements, you have always, in the last resort, to go outside the system itself, and take into account its relation to the rest of the whole system.... And for that very reason no subordinate individual, considered in itself, is a completely coherent self-determined whole."[15]

The viewpoint of the organicists once again can be explained in terms of the interrelated entities A, B, and C. Because they are interrelated to form a whole, the natures of these three entities are determined, at least in part, by the relational qualities they possess as parts of the whole. If A, for example, were considered in isolation from the whole, its true nature could not be determined because it would no longer have the relational properties it possessed when part of the whole. In fact, to be consistent an organicist would have to maintain that if A were taken from the whole it would be not-A, and the whole also would change.

McTaggart explains the matter in more detail: "Let us

take X, Y, and Z as representing all the infinite number of qualities possessed by some substance A, including those which are derivative from the relations in which A stands. . . . If now we enquire what A is, a complete answer must be given by giving the nature of A, and this consists of its qualities. X, Y, and Z are taken as a complete list of these, and thus the nature of A is X, Y, Z. Let us suppose any of the qualities altered, either by addition or subtraction or substitution, so that the complete list would be represented by W, X, Y, Z, or by X, Y, or by W, X, Y. Thus the nature of the substance which had such qualities would be different from the nature of A. Therefore the substance in question could not be A."[16]

The nature of A, then, cannot be determined by studying A apart. But there was more to the organicists' position than this: they also seemed to believe that when an entity was considered apart from the whole, it was not possible to predict what changes would take place (in the entity or in the whole) if the entity were incorporated into the whole.[17]

The organicists' position here can be attacked on several grounds. The major fault was pointed out earlier in the discussion of internal relations: the organicists held that *all* the characteristics of an entity determine its nature; in other words, all characteristics are defining characteristics. If this view is rejected—if it is held that only *some* characteristics of an entity are defining characteristics—the force of the organicists' fourth point disappears. For it then becomes apparent that at least some entities can be separated from the systems to which they belong without being altered in their natures; i.e. the defining characteristics of these entities are unaffected by the separation. It would therefore be possible to determine the nature of such entities by studying them in isolation.

The organicists were also assuming that one cannot predict, knowing that an entity has properties X, Y, and Z in isolation, what properties it will have when it comes into relationships with other entities. This assumption is unwarranted, and the organicists offer no evidence to show that this type of prediction is impossible. Moreover, the weight of the evidence is actually against the organicists here, for the physical sciences can provide numerous examples of successful prediction of the properties an entity will display when placed in novel conditions.*

The fifth constituent idea of organicism was stated as: "The parts are dynamically interrelated or interdependent." The entities A, B, and C, as parts of a whole, are interrelated; as a result, according to the theory of internal relations, the natures of B and C are in part determined by their relationship to A. Thus any change in A will change B and C, and the whole itself will also be changed. This is what organicists have referred to as the "dynamic" interrelationship of parts. Upon examination, however, there is nothing in this aspect of organicism that is incompatible with mechanism.

---

* For example, it is possible to predict the tensile strength of a plastic cord under extreme temperatures, or the resistance characteristics of an electrical component when placed in a given circuit.

It is apparent from the foregoing discussion that the five basic ideas of organicism, or Holism 1, are closely related. In fact, all five are based on the theory of internal relations; and modern organicism is, in a sense, no more than the Hegelian theory of internal relations writ large.

2

Organicism and Biology

IN THE LAST quarter of the nineteenth century, when neo-Hegelianism was the predominant school of philosophy in the English-speaking world, the analytic method was facing yet another severe trial. There was a marked reaction against it in the biological sciences, and, not surprisingly, Holism 1 was prominent in the dispute. The objection was not simply to the materialistic and antireligious nature of mechanistic analysis; rather, a number of developments in biology itself seemed to cast doubt on the feasibility of providing mechanistic explanations. In other words, it was being suggested in the second half of the nineteenth century that the concepts and methods used by adherents of the analytic approach were not capable of explaining the new discoveries in biology—a claim that is still echoed today. The history of late nineteenth-century biology is thus important to an understanding of twentieth-century holism.

Perhaps the chief difficulty concerned the theory of evolution. The Mendelian, or particulate, theory of heredity through discrete genes came in vogue only in the twentieth century, after Mendel's work was rediscovered; during the last decades of the nineteenth century a "blending" theory was favored. It was accepted that the spontaneous variations occurring in particular members of a species would tend to be blended or "diluted" as the variant individuals interbred with the nonvariants. It was difficult for the supporters of mechanistic analysis to explain how this blending or diluting of variations could allow evolutionary change to take place in a species; but an explanation could apparently be given by theories postulating the existence of a "life force" or a "creative urge" within individual organisms.[1] This apparent failure of the mechanistic explanation of evolution, and the success of the antimechanistic and antianalytic view, had important repercussions. Biologists were obsessed by the theory of evolution during these years, and the failure of mechanistic analysis to cope with this theory raised doubts about its effectiveness in other branches of the science.

One study affected was cellular biology. By the 1870's and 1880's it had become evident that earlier theorists had oversimplified matters. Instead of being a simple, basic entity, the cell was discovered to be very complex internally; indeed, it seemed so complex that many scientists could imagine no possible mechanism to account for its workings. The intricacies of cell structure revealed by microscopy, the inner complexity of the nucleus, and the elaborate process of cell division all presented difficulties. It was a matter of faith with some men that mechanistic analysis would eventually reign supreme—

a faith that was eventually vindicated by the work of Crick and Watson—but there were those who could not admit as feasible the degree of complexity that would be required by any conceivable mechanisms within each single cell.

The negative view persisted well into the new century, and as late as 1929 the biologist-philosopher J. S. Haldane could write: "The substance of cells must, on the mechanistic interpretation, be enormously complex and yet perfectly definite in molecular structure. But if it is so complex, how can we imagine it dividing into two parts? ... the more we ponder over this question the more clearly does it appear that the idea of a complex mechanism which can also reproduce itself or mend itself is not a coherent idea at all. In fact no scholastic absurdity was ever more of an absurdity."[2]

Difficulties for the opponents of holism were also raised by the behavior of cells in embryos. Experiments carried out on developing embryos around the turn of the century seemed to show that when an embryo had a section removed, its development altered so as to nullify, as far as possible, the effects of the damage. It seemed incomprehensible that any mechanism could account for this behavior in the embryo cells.[3]

One of the most important problems raised by the cell theory was itself not unrelated to the holistic question. In a multicellular organism, was each cell the unit of life, or was the whole organism in some way the unit? As the nineteenth century progressed, this came more and more under discussion. Many answers were forthcoming, but serious problems remained. Rudolf Virchow wrote in 1855, "Life is cell activity; its uniqueness is the uniqueness of the cell."[4] If so, how is the individuality or "oneness" of the whole organism produced? What enables the cells to cooperate? If, however, the cells are not the units, but the organism is still in some sense a whole, what produces this? What is the nature of the wholeness? Supporters of the mechanistic method were unable to answer these questions.

The reaction against mechanistic analysis in biology took a number of forms. To begin with, there was a resurgence of vitalism, supported by many arguments but especially by those intended to resolve the difficulties raised by evolutionary theory and cellular biology. Hans Driesch, in the forefront of the revival, postulated the existence within living things of a unifying factor or vital spirit, which he called the entelechy (borrowing the Aristotelian term). It was this entelechy that accounted for the surprising behavior of developing embryos, Driesch argued.

The vitalists were soon forced into an odd position. They had to postulate not only an entelechy within each cell but also a "master" entelechy belonging to the organism as a whole. Worse, they had to grant that the cellular entelechies themselves divided when the cells divided.[5] They never did decide how the master entelechy supposedly functioned, or how it was affected by the individual cells and their particular entelechies. The vitalistic position also suffered from the serious disadvantage that it tried to explain every life process as an

action of the entelechy, and thus it lost predictive power
—it was "a quite unsatisfactory hypothesis, both ultimately and from the standpoint of scientific advance."[6]

Related to vitalism was a second form of reaction to
mechanistic analysis, the theory of creative evolution. Its
proponents held that the life forces within living organisms were driving them onward, making them develop
into new forms. Thus evolution was creative, but the
cause of the creation lay within the organisms rather
than outside them, as the theory of natural selection had
postulated. Creative evolution seemed to provide an
escape from the difficulty faced by the combination of
evolutionary theory and the idea of blending heredity.
Samuel Butler supported one theory of creative evolution; variations were put forward in other contexts by
Henri Bergson (in *Creative Evolution*) and George
Bernard Shaw (in *Back to Methuselah*).

Yet another form of reaction was organicism. The biological organicists, as they shall be called, relied on the
holistic ideas of organicism discussed earlier. They insisted, for example, that "the physicochemical description of the vital processes does not exhaust them."[7] The
brothers R. B. and J. S. Haldane, writing in 1883, made
use of other organismic ideas: "It would thus appear
that the parts of an organism cannot be considered
simply as so many independent units, which happen to
be aggregated in a system in which each determines the
other. It is on the contrary the essential feature of each
part that it is a member of an ideal whole, which can
only be defined by saying that it realized itself in its

parts, and that the parts are only what they are insofar as they realize it."[8]

In 1884 J. S. Haldane contributed an article to *Mind* in which organismic ideas are readily detectable. His basic theme was that "the ordinary conceptions of physical science are insufficient when applied to the phenomena of life, and that other conceptions must be substituted."[9] In other words, Haldane was concerned with the first of the five constituent ideas of Holism 1, the idea that the analytic method (in the sense discussed earlier) was inadequate when applied to organic wholes. To illustrate his point, he cited two examples: the burrowing behavior of certain worms, which modify their activities in accordance with variations in the shape of objects they are dragging into their burrows; and the regeneration of the amputated legs of newts. These phenomena, Haldane wrote, "cannot be due to the mere action of neuro-muscular or intracellular mechanisms."[10]

Haldane's suggestion was that the notions of cause and effect are inadequate when applied to a living system. Rather than acting as cause and effect, the processes occurring in a living organism reciprocally determine each other; each part of an organic system is determined "through and through" by its interaction with the other parts of the whole. This is clearly the concept that has been presented here as the fifth constituent idea of organicism: the parts are dynamically interrelated or interdependent.

Haldane also accepted the third idea of organicism, for he went on to argue: "There is nothing in the parts that is not a manifestation of the whole. . . . In all that the parts do and all that they are they only show forth the whole. It follows from this that if we speak of them as determined by the whole, we use the word 'determined' in a sense altogether different from its ordinary sense. For, since the parts are what they are, only as taking part in the whole, there can clearly be nothing foreign to them in their determination. In this apparent determination they are only manifesting what they are in themselves."[11]

A detailed critique of Haldane's views will not be attempted here, for the points made would merely be repetitions of the criticisms already applied to Holism 1. However, it should be emphasized that the two concrete examples cited by Haldane would present no insurmountable difficulties for adherents of the analytic method. True, at the time Haldane was writing it was not possible to give an analytical explanation of the cases he brought forward. This was not a logical impossibility, however, but simply a practical impossibility in view of the relatively undeveloped state of the biological sciences at that time. Haldane, though, seems to have believed that it was in fact a logical impossibility—that his paper was clearly demonstrating the inherent shortcomings of mechanistic or analytic explanations in dealing with organic systems.

Another biological organicist of the late nineteenth century was Edmund Montgomery, who has recently been called a "pioneer of organicism."[12] Montgomery supported organicism in a number of technical biological papers, as well as in two more general essays published in *Mind*. In "The Unity of the Organic Individual" (1880) he mentioned his studies of cells and presented his conclusion that the fundamental entity was not the individual cell, but the organism as a whole: "The distinct morphological divisions of higher animals are indeed integrant, not constituent, parts. They are specialized and segregated from a pre-existing whole, and are in no way discrete and independent units joined together in the composition of a complex totality.... The whole is here in all reality antecedent to its parts. The organism is prior to its tissues, the tissues prior to their supposed elements. The centralised organism is not, as universally assumed, a multiple of ultimate units, but is, on the contrary, itself one single individuality."[18]

Thus the biological organicists believed that the processes occurring in living things could be understood only when the features of the whole organism were considered. The organism was a functioning unit, and it was this unit that determined the characteristics of the constituent parts, not vice versa. A piecemeal examination of the parts, they were suggesting, would not bring understanding of the whole.

Another line of development followed by biological organicism in the decades after 1880 was an extension of the idea of wholeness such that the whole, the functioning unit, became not the organism itself but the organism together with its environment. J. S. Haldane, for example, wrote: "These parts [of the organism] stand to one another, and to the surroundings, not in the relation of cause and effect but in that of reciprocity. *The parts of an organism and its surroundings thus form a system,* any one of the parts of which constantly acts on the rest, but only does so, *qua* part of the system, insofar as they at the same time act on it."[14]

It was here that the ideas of the biological organicists approached those of the neo-idealists. The point is that if the whole is the organism plus the environment, then, because there is no boundary in nature separating an organism's environment from the rest of the universe, the planet Mars, Mount Everest, and every other entity are all part of the environment of any and every biological organism. And if it is held that the parts can only be understood in relation to the whole, then the attainment of knowledge becomes impossible. Once again we have the situation presented by Russell: "If all knowledge were knowledge of the universe as a whole, there would be no knowledge."

Beginning about 1880, biological organicism reached its peak in the twentieth century; and among the biologists writing from this perspective in the early 1900's were J. S. Haldane, J. H. Woodger, C. Lloyd Morgan, E. R. Russell, and W. E. Agar. There were also influential supporters outside biology—the statesman Jan Christian Smuts and the philosopher A. N. Whitehead, to mention two. But from about 1930 biological organicism began to take on new dimensions, and became something beyond a mere group of five interrelated holistic theses set in opposition to the analytic method.

3

Reductionism, Individuals, and Systems

DURING THE 1920's and 1930's, two young Continental biologists, Paul Weiss and Ludwig von Bertalanffy, were thinking along similar lines; and their later careers in some ways continued on parallel courses. Both reached eminence in their respective fields, both became professors in North America, and both maintained a common core of ideas related to holism. Weiss, especially, has been a consistent critic of the limitations of what he calls "the method of analytical decomposition," and some of his more recent papers illustrate the advances that have been made over the biological organicism of the late nineteenth century.

To state the central issues briefly at the outset, what seems to have happened in Weiss's work is that other holistic theses, here termed *Holism 2* and *Holism 3*, were linked with Holism 1 (or organicism). But this linkage was obscured, first, by the fact that the added theses tended to resemble some of the five basic ideas that constitute Holism 1 and hence were easily confused with them. To complicate matters, Weiss wrote as if he was defending only one cause instead of many; and he admitted outright that the analytic method had its uses and was compatible with some of what he was advocating (his position, as he saw it, was more a reconciliation between the dogmas of mechanism and holism than a replacement for mechanism). Finally, even within a single paper he treated "analytical decomposition" as first one concept and then another; but he appeared not to recognize that the two concepts were quite different, and regarded them merely as alternative statements of a central mechanistic, analytic, or reductionist thesis.

All this is not to deny the pertinence of much of Weiss's position, nor to suggest that he is a solitary figure. At an interdisciplinary conference in 1968, several prominent scholars in related fields (including Bertalanffy) put forward similar cases and specifically endorsed Weiss's arguments.[1] And as we shall see, he also had precursors among philosophers and social scientists earlier in the century.

It is useful at the outset to consider a passage from Weiss's fascinating paper "$1 + 1 \neq 2$ (One Plus One Does Not Equal Two)": "Specifically, these are the points I aim to prove: (1) that as our brain scans features of the universe we shift range and focus back and forth between telescopic and microscopic vision, as it were; (2) that as we move downward on this scale, we mostly gain precision and lose perspective; (3) that as we move upward, new and relevant features, formerly unrecognizable and unsuspected, come into view; (4) that this emerging novelty pertains to macro-samples of nature—

that is, that it reflects properties of collectives—of groups, assemblies, systems, and populations, composed of microsamples; and (5) that the required additional terms to characterize such collectives must come from rigorous scientific procedure rather than from anthropomorphic translocations and allegorical allusions to mythology."[2]

These, in abbreviated form, are Weiss's main contentions; and the passage can be used to illustrate the general points made earlier in this chapter. In the first place, it is evident that Weiss saw shortcomings in the analytic method. "As we move downward" along the path cleared by analysis, "we mostly gain precision and lose perspective." Elsewhere in the same paper his classical organicism came even more into the open. "Let us ask first: Of what do we deprive a system when we dismember it and isolate its component parts, whether bodily or just in our mind? Plainly, of the *interrelations* that had existed among the parts while they were still united."[3] Sometimes Weiss gave his case more contemporary impact by arguing that what is lost in the process of analysis is "information content." This was still a form of Holism 1, for the basis of his rejection of analysis as a suitable method of investigation was the existence of interrelationships between the parts of an organic whole.

To return to the passage first quoted: it can be seen that Weiss immediately connected Holism 1 with a somewhat different thesis, namely, that as "we move upward" we find cases of the "unsuspected," of "emerging novelty"; in other words, the phenomenon of emergence. Taken at face value, this could simply be a restatement of one of the five basic ideas of organicism, "the whole is more than the sum of the parts." But other passages suggest that Weiss was taking the argument beyond this. The extension is indicated by his not infrequent use of the term "reductionism" when referring to the analytic method. It is one thing to argue that *as a method of working*, analysis has shortcomings; it is another to argue that from knowledge of the parts *only* —that is, in the absence of any knowledge of the whole— the emergent properties of the whole cannot be predicted (but both of these are part of the organicists' credo). However, it is quite different from both of these to maintain that *after* knowledge of the whole has somehow been obtained, *then* this cannot be reduced to (i.e. explained in terms of) the properties and "summation" of the parts. It is this last thesis that a reductionist would oppose, for he believes the properties can be so reduced.

In taking this position the reductionist is arguing not against Holism 1 but against Holism 2. Weiss gave a forthright account of Holism 2 and its antireductionism: "To explain life, static cell anatomy must become molecular ecology, organisms be comprehended through cell ecology, and societies through the dynamics of human ecology. They all provide us with examples of rigorous scientific propositions that hold for groups but dissolve when efforts are made to reduce them to elemental properties. Here resolution becomes sheer dissolution."[4]

It is worth stressing this important distinction. Holism 1 maintains, in part, that if one has knowledge of the

[33]

parts only, then at least some properties of organic wholes or systems cannot be predicted. To revert to the simple chemical example used earlier, if one knew only the properties of hydrogen and oxygen from studying them separately and in isolation, then it could not be predicted that when combined they would form the (emergent) colorless, odorless, and tasteless liquid water. By contrast, Holism 2 maintains that the properties of organic wholes or systems, *after* they have been found, cannot be explained in terms of the properties of the parts. This is analogous to arguing (although holists would not use this example) that when the properties of water have been ascertained, they cannot then be accounted for in terms of the properties and "summation" of hydrogen and oxygen.

It will be shown in some detail later on that Holism 2 has had a prominent position in the social sciences; it is sufficient at this stage to illustrate Paul Weiss's adherence to the thesis: "So, here I have at last put my finger on the sore spot, the touching of which has for ages hurt the protagonists of analytical-reductionist orthodoxy— the concept of *wholeness*. Refusing to look beyond their ultimate and most extreme abstraction, namely, the presumption of truly 'isolated' elements in nature, *and spurred by the dramatic success of explanations of many complex effects in terms of interactions among such elements*, they could not help but ask what there could be then in the universe other than elements and interactions."[5]

Having offered this somewhat hostile but fairly accurate sketch of the reductionist view, Weiss went on to point out that in nature there are "ordered complexes." But here he made a serious mistake, for he thought he was arguing against reductionism when he stated that these complexes must be studied before they could be explained: "The empirical dichotomy arises between *simple conglomerates* and the type of ordered complexes which we designate as systems. In other words, systems are products of our experience with nature, and not mental constructs, and whoever without being privy to that primary practical experience would try to abrogate them, could do so only by arrogation."[6] As has been pointed out, the reductionist does not necessarily disagree with this. Weiss was confusing the opponents of Holism 1 with those of Holism 2.

To return once more to the original quotation: Weiss can be seen to move through Holisms 1 and 2 to reach still another position, namely, that "additional terms" are required "to characterize such collectives." Elsewhere he argues, "What the task calls for is, first of all, a job of thorough conceptual overhauling and renovation."[7] One characteristic of Weiss's papers is the range of biological examples that he uses; consequently, his case for the use of such holistic concepts as that of "hierarchies" is indeed impressive. But of course the thesis that there is an important place in science for concepts referring to properties of wholes—a thesis that can be called Holism 3—is one that supporters of the analytic method and of reductionism can both endorse.

Neither analytic nor reductionist science opposes conceptual advance and renovation. In physics, for example, where both these positions are firmly entrenched, many new concepts have been introduced over the years, including ones that relate to Holism 3 (e.g. the concepts pertaining to field theory). To use an earlier example, it has long been recognized that water, the whole, has properties markedly different from those of its constituent elements, hydrogen and oxygen. It is not unheard of for scientists to introduce new concepts in order to facilitate their investigation of such emergent properties. This in no way contradicts the reductionist thesis that the properties of the whole, however they are described, are explicable in terms of the properties and "summation" of constituent elements.

Weiss, then, was wrong to summarize his attack on reductionism in these words: "I herewith rest my case. Biology has made spectacular advances by adopting the disciplined methods of the inorganic sciences and mathematics, but it has not widened its conceptual framework in equal measure. My aim was to illustrate not only the need, but the flexibility of such an adaptive move."[8] To assert Holism 3, as Weiss does here, is not to attack reductionism at all.

The situation may be briefly summarized:

Holism 1, the five theses of organicism; opposed by supporters of the analytic/mechanistic method, who nonetheless accept several of the organismic theses.

Holism 2 states that a whole, even after it is studied, cannot be explained in terms of its parts; opposed by reductionism.

Holism 3 states that it is necessary to have terms referring to wholes and their properties; also acceptable to supporters of the analytic method and reductionism.

The discussion of Weiss's biological papers has prepared the way for a consideration of numerous similar arguments that have been applied to material closer to the interests of social scientists—namely, those arguments that form the core of the controversy between methodological holists and methodological individualists in sociology, anthropology, and history. Both positions in this dispute have a long and complex history, with the result—common in such cases—that it is difficult to arrive at a clear and simple statement that the disputants agree gives a fair picture of the central issues.

A passage from one of the classic sources, Emile Durkheim's *The Rules of Sociological Method* (1895), at least offers a reasonable starting point: "At the same time that it is teleological, the method of explanation generally followed by sociologists is essentially psychological. These two tendencies are interconnected with one another. In fact, if society is only a system of means instituted by men to attain certain ends, these ends can only be individual, for only individuals could have existed before society. From the individual, then, have emanated the needs and desires determining the formation of societies; and if it is from him that all comes, it is necessarily by him that all must be explained.... Hence, sociological laws can be only a corollary of the more general laws of psychology; the ultimate explanation of collective life will consist in showing how it emanates from human nature in general."[9]

The position outlined here—and later attacked by Durkheim—was methodological individualism. It is apparent that, as J. W. N. Watkins has emphasized, this position is analogous to mechanism, that is, to the view that "the ultimate constituents of the physical world are impenetrable particles which obey simple mechanical laws."[10] For methodological individualism holds that every "complex social situation, institution, or event is the result of a particular configuration of individuals, their dispositions, situations, beliefs, and physical resources and environment."[11] In other words, the central thesis of methodological individualism appears to be a form of reductionism, and is therefore in opposition to Holism 2 but not to Holisms 1 or 3 (notwithstanding the fact that many individualists have been, on other grounds, also opposed to most of the ideas that constitute Holism 1).

Although there have been innumerable variations and subtleties in the arguments against methodological individualism, all three forms of holism have made an appearance, and they have been confused and intertwined in much the same way as they were in the writings of Paul Weiss.

To find an example of Holism 1, or organicism, one has only to return to the work of Durkheim. After outlining individualism in the terms quoted earlier, he developed his attack on it along the following lines. Individualism fails because society is not "merely an extension of the individual being";[12] society exerts "pressure" on individuals, thereby showing that it has powers not possessed by the individual. "This pressure," Durkheim states, "is the pressure which the totality exerts on the individual." His next words give a clear statement of several organismic theses: "But, it will be said that, since the only elements making up society are individuals, the first origins of sociological phenomena cannot but be psychological. In reasoning thus, it can be established just as easily that organic phenomena may be explained by inorganic phenomena. It is very certain that there are in the living cell only molecules of crude matter. But these molecules are in contact with one another, and this association is the cause of the new phenomena which characterize life, the very germ of which cannot possibly be found in any of the separate elements. A whole is not identical with the sum of its parts. It is something different, and its properties differ from those of its component parts."[13]

Evidently, Durkheim was attempting to combat methodological individualism not with the Holism 2 that was in opposition to it, but with Holism 1. The individualist typically argues that social phenomena can be reduced to—that is, explained in terms of—the characteristics and behavior (including its unforeseen consequences) of individuals, whereas the adherent of Holism 2 argues for irreducibility. The individualist is not bound to come out in opposition to one constituent idea of Holism 1 and hold that emergent or "new" phenomena can be predicted beforehand on the basis of knowledge of the elements. Certainly the "germ" of the "new phenomena" may not be discernible in advance in the separate elements, and individualists such as Popper and Watkins, in their attacks on historicist prediction, frequently pointed to this kind of difficulty in the social sciences. They were not contradicting this aspect of Holism 1, which was central to Durkheim's argument, when they insisted: "There may be unfinished or half-way explanations of large-scale social phenomena (say, inflation) in terms of other large-scale phenomena (say, full employment); but we shall not have arrived at rock-bottom explanations of such large-scale phenomena until we have deduced an account of them from statements about the dispositions, beliefs, resources and interrelations of individuals."[14]

It is only Holism 2 that is directly opposed to methodological individualism. Maurice Mandelbaum seems to have recognized this, and in his paper "Societal Facts" he argued for irreducibility: "My aim is to show that one cannot understand the actions of human beings as members of a society unless one assumes that there is a group of facts which I shall term 'societal facts' which are as ultimate as are those facts which are 'psychological' in character ... those concepts which are used to refer to the forms of organization of a society cannot be reduced without remainder to concepts which only refer to the thoughts and actions of specific individuals."[15]

The main argument here is that in attempting to replace a societal fact by facts about individuals, some other societal concepts will have to be used. This is what Mandelbaum means by saying it is impossible to effect a reduction "without remainder." Thus, if we tried to explain in individualistic terms the behavior of a bank teller—why he adopts a certain role, why a slip of paper (a check or withdrawal form) presented by a customer can move him to action, and so on—we would run into difficulty. Our individualistic argument might claim that he acts as he does in reaction to the way other individuals act toward him. But why does he only react to certain people (customers, or the bank manager, but not friends at a party), and why is it that customers treat him the way they do? As Mandelbaum put it, "We have seen in the foregoing illustration that my own behavior toward the bank teller is determined by his status. If the attempt is now made to interpret his status in terms of the recurrent patterns of behavior which others exemplify in dealing with him, then their behavior is left unexplained; each of them—no less than I—will only behave in this way because each recognizes the teller of the bank to have a particular status."[16]

Watkins replied to this line of argument by pointing out that Mandelbaum was discussing the irreducibility of societal *facts*, whereas the interesting issue, and the one most individualists were concerned with, was whether there were irreducible societal *laws*. Watkins's pertinent remarks were contained in a footnote, so his case was not developed at any length. But he did state: "An individualist may readily admit . . . that some large social facts are simply too complex for a full reduction of them to be feasible, and yet hold that individualistic explanations of them are in principle possible."[17]

The chemical analogy used earlier in discussing the arguments of Paul Weiss may also be useful here. The facts about the behavior of the chemical compound water, and in particular its reactions with other compounds, may be too complex to describe in the terminology of atoms (the properties and behavior of hydrogen and oxygen atoms and the constituents of the other relevant compounds); and in fact new terminology ("colorless, odorless, tasteless liquid" or something similar) may have been introduced specifically to facilitate discussion of the emergent properties of water and these other compounds. But this does not mean that precise explanations of the behavior of water in terms of the characteristics of atoms and the laws applicable to them will not be forthcoming. In fact, it could be argued that modern valency theory provides a means for giving such explanations.

Another defense against Mandelbaum's attack was developed by Joseph Agassi, who stressed that the individualist does not deny either that " 'society' affects the individual's aims (collectivism)" or that the "social set-up influences and constrains the individual's behavior (institutional analysis)."[18] It is only when these two principles are "reinterpreted" in the light of a false holistic principle—"if 'wholes' exist *then* they have distinct aims and interests of their own"—that the individualist becomes opposed to them. To revert to Mandelbaum's example, the individualist does not deny that the behavior of the bank teller and his customers is influenced by the social situation in which they find themselves.

Agassi's argument highlights the individualist's rejection of even the vaguest suggestion that "social entities" exist in the same way that individuals do; and analysis of the writings of Watkins and F. A. von Hayek confirms this. Consider first the words of Hayek, who wrote of "methodological collectivism" as the "tendency to treat 'wholes' like 'society' or the 'economy,' 'capitalism' (as a given historical 'phase') or a particular 'industry' or 'class' or 'country' as definitely given objects about which we can discover laws by observing their behavior as wholes."[19] Hayek's subsequent argument was that these social entities were not "given to observation" but instead resulted from the application of a theory. Social scientists may postulate, or even think they see, the existence of a business firm; but what they have actually done is construct a model "to explain the connection between some of the individual phenomena" they have observed.[20]

Watkins at one point suggested that holism might be regarded as the view in which "some superhuman agents or factors are supposed to be at work in history."[21] In another essay he insisted that human societies are not organisms even in the somewhat restricted sense that a community of social insects might be labeled with that term: "The principle whose status I have been trying to elucidate is a methodological rule which presupposes the factual assertion that human social systems are not organisms in the above sense."[22]

[43]

This passage is also of interest because of Watkins's characterization of individualism as a *methodological rule*. A rule, of course, is neither true nor false but is judged by its fruitfulness. Is individualism, then, a fruitful approach to the human sciences? One relevant point arises immediately: however many the advantages of the holistic position, the individualistic approach must have even more; for the individualist can accept most, if not all, of what the holist uncovers in the course of his investigations, but the individualist will then press on to attempt a reduction.

The foregoing discussion should have suggested that although individualists have been firmly opposed to Holism 2 (and usually to some of the constituent ideas of Holism 1), they have had no objection to Holism 3. Terminology that refers to "social wholes" has been acceptable, but the methodological individualist has always added that "all social phenomena, and especially the functioning of all social institutions, should always be understood as resulting from the decisions, actions, attitudes, etc., of human individuals.... *We should never be satisfied by an explanation in terms of so-called 'collectives.'* "[23]

Like Paul Weiss and the methodological holists, Ludwig von Bertalanffy also grappled with the phenomenon of organic wholeness. He, too, was trained as a biologist, and in *Modern Theories of Development* (1933), a work centering around the problems of embryology, he wrote: "Mechanism ... provides us with no grasp of the specific characteristics of organisms, of the organization of organic processes among one another, of organic 'wholeness,' of the problem of the origin of organic 'teleology,' or of the historical character of organisms. . . . We must therefore try to establish a new standpoint which—as opposed to mechanism—takes account of organic wholeness, but . . . treats it in a manner which admits of scientific investigation."[24]

Later Bertalanffy called again for the full and rigorous development of the holistic view (at this stage he was no more specific), for he had the fervent belief of a prophet that such a view would throw light not only on biological systems but on *all* systems: "From the statement we have made, a stupendous perspective emerges, a vista towards a hitherto unsuspected unity of the conception of the world. Similar general principles have evolved everywhere, whether we are dealing with inanimate things, organisms, mental or social processes. What is the origin of these correspondences? We answer this question by the claim for a new realm of science, which we call General System Theory. It is a logico-mathematical field, the subject matter of which is the formulation and derivation of those principles which hold for systems in general. A 'system' can be defined as a complex of elements standing in interaction. There are general principles holding for systems, irrespective of the nature of the component elements and of the relations or forces between them."[25] In 1948, at Alpbach, Bertalanffy publicly launched this General System Theory.[26]

4

The Bases of General System Theory

THE PROOF for the existence of God that has become known as the ontological proof has the interesting characteristic that at one moment it can command assent whereas at the next it seems obviously invalid. This is illustrated by a story told of Bertrand Russell. Once, while rambling through the countryside with some friends, he was observed to come to a sudden stop and exclaim, "Good Lord! The ontological proof *is* valid!" Perhaps in future years similar stories will be told about system theory, for this possesses the same intriguing characteristic as the ontological proof. At times, a critical reader feels that what system theorists are saying is both important and true; on other occasions only the former judgment seems warranted.

The men who struggled to establish what after 1948 became recognizable as General System Theory were primarily concerned with the same methodological problem that occupied the organicists. This is no surprise, for system theory is actually another form of Holism 1. The problem, of course, was the most appropriate method of studying any organic whole or system. Ludwig von Bertalanffy has written of his realization during the 1930's that the traditional methods of science "had proved insufficient to deal with theoretical problems, especially in the biosocial sciences."[1] And in 1969 he wrote: " 'Analytical procedure' means that an entity investigated be resolved into, and hence can be constituted or reconstituted from, the parts put together. . . . This is the basic principle of 'classical' science, which can be circumscribed in different ways: resolution into isolable causal trains, seeking for 'atomic' units in the various fields of science, etc. The progress of science has shown that these principles of classical science—first enunciated by Galileo and Descartes—are highly successful in a wide realm of phenomena."[2]

But system theorists, like the organicists, go on to claim that there is a certain "realm of phenomena" where the analytic method is not successful—phenomena involving what they variously describe as "wholes," "organized complexities," or "systems." They repeat the now familiar argument that these have a logical structure that makes the analytic method inappropriate; what is required is a new approach, and it is this that the system theorists claim to have provided in General System Theory (or GST): "General system theory, therefore, is a general science of 'wholeness' which up till now was considered a vague, hazy, and semi-metaphysical concept. In elaborate form it would be a logico-mathematical discipline, in itself purely formal but applicable to the various empirical sciences. For sciences concerned

with 'organized wholes,' it would be of similar significance to that which probability theory has for sciences
concerned with 'chance events'; the latter, too, is a formal mathematical discipline which can be applied to the
most diverse fields, such as thermodynamics, biological
and medical experimentation, genetics, life insurance
statistics, etc."[3]

The foregoing discussion will serve as an introduction
to General System Theory. In the following pages four
features of GST have been selected for examination:
(1) the failure of system theorists to sustain their methodological objections to the analytic method; (2) the
failure to specify precisely what is meant by a "system";
(3) the vagueness over what is to be included within
system theory; (4) the failure of GST as a scientific
theory.

1. *The failure of system theorists to sustain their methodological objections to the analytic method.* In order
to evaluate the sweeping claims made for GST it is necessary to examine once again the structure of "wholes" or
"systems." The peculiarity of systems that is held to make
the analytic method an inappropriate one for studying
them is that *they have parts that cannot be meaningfully
separated from each other*—a point that has emerged in
previous chapters. The parts of a mechanical device or
"aggregate"—e.g. a motor or a clock—can be separated
from each other and studied in mutual isolation without
destroying anything essential to their natures; hence a
spark plug can be removed from an engine without destroying any essential characteristic that the plug posses-

ses. But the parts of a biological, political, or business system cannot be separated from each other without destroying something essential. For it is claimed that by their very nature all parts of such systems are inextricably related to each other; and by separating the parts of a system in order to study them in isolation, we are actually destroying the parts and creating artifacts.

As A. Angyal put the point in 1941, paralleling one of the key arguments of Holism 1, "It should also be kept in mind that 'part' means something different when applied to aggregate from what it means when applied to wholes. When the single objects a, b, c, d are bound together in an aggregate they participate in that aggregation as object a, object b, object c, etc., that is, as lines, distances, color spots, or whatever they may be. When, however, a whole is constituted by the utilization of objects a, b, c, d, the parts of the resulting whole are *not* object a, object b, object c, etc., but a, β, γ, δ."[4] Thus, if part a is moved from the system or whole for examination in isolation, it is no longer a, for it is no longer related to the other parts; the act of removing a changes it, and it becomes artifact a.

It was pointed out earlier that this line of argument advanced by the system theorists was not a product of the mid-twentieth century; an identical position was held by Hegel and his followers, but instead of calling it "system theory" they gave it the title "principle of internal or organic relations." The American philosopher John Dewey (1859–1952) was educated in this Hegelian tradition, and later in his life he admitted that his acquaintance with Hegel's philosophy had left a permanent mark on his own thought. Some of Dewey's work, with its strong Hegelian overtones, must count as a direct contribution to contemporary system theory.[5] In particular, during the 1940's Dewey collaborated with Arthur F. Bentley in writing a series of articles (which eventually became a book, *Knowing and the Known*) to discuss the same problem of relations that lies at the heart of system theory. But only Bentley has received a passing brief reference in Bertalanffy's *General System Theory*.

Dewey's involvement with the problem of relations long antedates Bertalanffy's. In his writings on the philosophical problem of knowledge, Dewey had run into problems with terminology; he argued that there was no term in the traditional philosophical vocabulary to express what he believed to be the true nature of the relation between the knower and the environment about which knowledge was sought. In 1917, in his essay "The Need for a Recovery of Philosophy" in *Creative Intelligence*, he referred to the knowing organism as an "agent-patient"—the organism was both affecting and being affected by the environment, and it was an error to study the organism in isolation. Even earlier, in 1884, he had written: "The idea of environment is a necessity to the idea of organism, and with the conception of environment comes the impossibility of considering psychical life as an individual, isolated thing developing in a vacuum."[6] Dewey, then, was close to the view that the organism and its environment form a system. Later, during the 1930's, he used the terms "transaction" and "situation" to express his view of the relation between an organism and its environment, and between the knower and the world around him.

Perhaps Dewey's most important discussions of the nature of relations are to be found in the articles he wrote with Bentley. The two started from the position that Dewey, at least, had adopted before the turn of the century. They accepted that man was an organism produced in the course of evolution, and hence that all of man's "behavings" were not activities "of himself alone" but were "processes of the full situation of organism-environment."[7] During the development of the human race in historical times, they argued, both the way in which men investigated nature and the way in which they reported the results of their investigations had undergone development through three stages (although Dewey and Bentley made the point that there were no clear-cut divisions between the stages).

These "three levels of the organization and presentation of inquiry" were, in historical order, the levels of self-action, of inter-action, and of trans-action.[8] (A contemporary system theorist would no doubt call these the level of self-action, the level of analytic or mechanical explanation, and the level of system theory.) Self-action, the most primitive level, was the level at which "things" were viewed as acting under their own power. Interaction was seen by Dewey and Bentley as the level "where thing is balanced against thing in causal interconnection." Trans-action was the level "where systems of description and naming are employed to deal with aspects and phrases of action, without final attribution to 'elements' or other presumptively detachable or independent 'entities,' 'essences,' or 'realities,' and without isolation of presumptively detachable 'relations' from such detachable 'elements.' "[9]

In the article "Interaction and Transaction," where these points were expounded, the authors argued that physical science was displaying a tendency to move away from the level of interactional systems of description (the type of description exemplified by the post-Newtonian science of mechanics, and the type for which the traditional analytic method is adequate), toward the transactional (or system) level. In another paper, "Transactions as Known and Named," they set out to show the increasing use of transactional explanations for "behavioral inquiry."[10] It was in this second article that Dewey and Bentley took up the issue of the method of studying relations in certain types of complex systems: "If interaction is procedure such that its inter-acting constituents are set up in inquiry as separate 'facts,' each in independence of the presence of others, then *Trans-action* is Fact such that no one of its constituents can be adequately specified as 'a fact' apart from the specification of the other constituents of the full subject matter."[11]

They went on to illustrate the differences between the inter-actional and trans-actional approaches by using the examples of a billiard game and a loan of money. The position of the balls on the table in a game of billiards can be studied inter-actionally, the two authors argued, but a wider, or "cultural," account of the game can only be given in trans-actional terms. And in the case of a loan of money, no words can be found to give a purely inter-actional account, since there are no "primarily separate items" that can be named in inter-actional terms. The authors went on: "Borrower cannot borrow without lender to lend, nor lender lend without borrower to borrow, the loan being a transaction that is identifiable only in the wider transaction of the full legal-commercial system in which it is present as event."[12]

In at least one respect the loan example was unfortunate. One of Dewey's philosophical mentors, William James, had been an outspoken critic of certain aspects of Hegel's philosophy, including the principle of internal relations that was reflected in Dewey's and Bentley's handling of the loan illustration. James, writing more than half a century before Dewey and Bentley and with his sights set on organicism rather than on system theory, had used a strikingly similar example to ridicule the very point that the later writers were making seriously: "It costs nothing, not even a mental effort, to admit that the absolute totality of things may be organized exactly after the pattern of one of these 'through-and-through' abstractions. In fact, it is the pleasantest and freest of mental movements. Husband makes, and is made by, wife, through marriage; one makes other by being itself other; everything is self-created through its opposite— you go round like a squirrel in a cage.... *What, in fact, is the logic of these abstract systems? It is, as we said above: if any Member, then the Whole System; if not the Whole System, then Nothing.*"[13]

Despite this historical irony, the example given by Dewey and Bentley does bring to the fore the central issue of system theory. It is a fact that in certain types of systems each part or element seems to take on its identity only by virtue of its relation to the others. If there is no borrower, then there can be no lender; and if there is a husband, then there must be a wife. But does it follow from this undeniable point that any such part cannot be taken and studied in isolation? Is it impossible to isolate, without distortion, the borrower from the lender who by giving him money also gives him his identity as a borrower, or the husband from the wife who has made him a husband? Dewey and Bentley had no doubts about the answer: "In ordinary, everyday behavior, in what sense can we examine a talking unless we bring a hearing along with it into account? Or a writing without a reading? Or a buying without a selling?"[14]

Bertalanffy would seem to have agreed: "Every organism represents a *system,* by which term we mean a complex of elements in mutual interaction. From this obvious statement the limitations of the analytical and summative conceptions must follow. First, it is impossible to resolve the phenomena of life completely into elementary units; for each individual part and each individual event depends not only on conditions within itself, but also to a greater or lesser extent on the conditions within the *whole*, or within superordinate units of which it is a part. Hence the behavior of an isolated part is, in general, different from its behavior within the context of the whole.... Secondly, the actual whole shows properties that are absent from its isolated parts."[15]

There are compelling reasons for believing that Hegel, Dewey, Bentley, the organicists, and the system theorists were and are mistaken. Borrowers, talkers, and husbands *can* be separated from their respective lenders, hearers, and wives, and can be meaningfully studied in isolation. Certainly a man cannot be directly studied in his role as a husband if he is isolated from his wife; this is a truism that can be recognized without the assistance of system theory. But even though he is isolated from his wife, he is the same man; personal identity does not depend on the possession of one characteristic alone. As argued earlier, a thing can still be the same thing when one of its characteristics is altered; for most characteristics are only accompanying characteristics, and furthermore most things are defined by reference to a cluster of characteristics, in which one or two characteristics can leave or join without the thing becoming different.[16] (It was these insights that were bound up, in philosophy, with the refutation of much of Hegel's work.)

Although a man's specific role as a husband cannot be studied directly when he is isolated, his many physical and intellectual features can be studied; the attitudes, expectations, and "world view" that help to shape his dealings with the world can be tested and measured; his socioeconomic status can be categorized; and his views about sex, family life, child nurture, and women's liberation can be recorded. These characteristics are not what make him a husband, but they are part of the cluster of characteristics that make him an individual. The knowledge of these characteristics gained by studying him in isolation from his wife will throw much light on what he is like in his role as a husband—it may even be possible, on the basis of this analytically derived information, to make accurate predictions about the characteristics he will display in this role. So it would appear that a great deal of reliable and relevant information can be ascertained by studying elements in isolation from the whole system.

Whether accurate predictions about the whole can be made on the basis of knowledge of the parts will depend on what laws and theories have been established in the field concerned. Ernest Nagel has argued forcefully that if such prediction is not possible at a given moment because those generalizations are lacking, this "does *not* mean that it is *in principle* impossible to explain such total behavior mechanistically, and it supplies no competent evidence for such a claim."[17] The good common sense of Dewey and Bentley led them to acknowledge something of this; but they did not appreciate that in doing so they had irretrievably weakened their case: "How can we have a principal without an agent or an agent without a principal? We can, of course, detach any portion of a transaction that we wish, and secure provisional descriptions and partial reports. But all this must be subject to the wider observation of the full process."[18]

The case for system theory rests to a large degree on the claim that a part cannot be removed from a system without becoming an artifact; it is fatal to ruin this foundation by admitting that useful information can be obtained by studying a part in isolation. And it does not save the case to argue, as Dewey and Bentley did, that the information so obtained "must be subject to the wider observation of the full process." It is almost another truism to assert that any predictions made about a man's performance as a husband on the basis of information gained by studying him in isolation will still have to be tested by studying him *as* a husband. And of course any predictions that are made about a whole complex economic system after studying only a few of its features cannot be checked unless the complete system is observed. Perhaps it is the presence of these truistic elements that gives system theory the enigmatic quality referred to at the beginning of this chapter.

The "loan of money" example used by Dewey and Bentley, and even more the "husband and wife" parody presented by William James, brings to light a further weakness that system theory shares with other forms of Holism 1. James had pointed out that the logic "of these abstract systems" was that in order to know anything about any member one must know everything about the whole. Accepting the theses of Holism 1, the adherents of system theory argue that the husband cannot be studied in isolation from the wife, or the wife in isolation from the husband; thus knowledge about a part can *only* be derived from knowledge of the whole.

Hence James's derision: this is an impossible methodology to work with, for *everything* would have to be known before *anything* could be known!

Examination of what the adherents of system theory actually do in practice bears out this analysis. Since the methodology they profess to accept is an impossible one, it is not surprising to find that they do not actually use it; that is, they do not first obtain knowledge of the whole and then derive from this some knowledge of the parts. As Ernest Nagel put the point in his discussion of systems ideas in biology (that is, organismic biology): "It is beyond serious question that advances in biology occur only through the use of an abstractive method, which proceeds to study various aspects of organic behavior in relative isolation of other aspects.... Organismic biologists proceed in this way, for they have no alternative. For example, in spite of his insistence on the indivisible unity of the organism, J. S. Haldane's work on respiration and the chemistry of the blood did not proceed by considering the body as a whole, but by studying the relations between the behavior of one part of the body ... and the behavior of another part."[19]

System theorists certainly do place great stress on interrelationships between parts, perhaps more than some (though by no means all) "traditional" scientists have done; but they do this by using techniques and concepts derived from traditional analytic science, such as flow charts and feedback diagrams, the concept of entropy, and the "principle of equifinality." A more detailed discussion of the application of system theory to the social sciences will be given in Chapter 5.

System theorists also make use of sophisticated mathematical techniques. In his *General System Theory*, Bertalanffy argues that the use of modern mathematics has led to the investigation of systems of great complexity; and that traditional mathematics could not cope with systems consisting of parts "in interaction" because "the prototype of their description is a set of simultaneous differential equations which are nonlinear in the general case."[20] If Bertalanffy's subsequent technical argument is sound, it establishes that certain newly available mathematical techniques for the first time *allow* certain systems to be investigated as wholes, in the sense that effects on the whole system of variations in one of the interrelated parts can be computed.

However, this argument does not establish either that systems *have* to be investigated as wholes in this way or that it is misguided to adopt an analytic or mechanistic approach. And Bertalanffy gives the game away by writing: "Naturally, an incongruence between model and reality often exists. There are highly elaborate and sophisticated mathematical models, but it remains dubious how they can be applied to the concrete case; there are fundamental problems for which no mathematical techniques are available. Disappointment of overextended expectations has occurred. Cybernetics, e.g., proved its impact ... but it did not yield an all-embracing explanation or grand world view, being an extension rather than a replacement of the mechanistic view and machine theory."[21] But there is a case for claiming that every method used by adherents of system theory *must* be "an extension rather than a replacement of the mechanistic view."

2. *The failure to specify precisely what is meant by a "system."* GST has as its purpose the formulation of laws applicable to all systems, irrespective of what actually composes the elements of these systems. Although somewhat ambitious, this quest is not necessarily quixotic; everything depends on what is meant by the term "system." But here again the accounts given by system theorists have been unsatisfactory.

Bertalanffy defined a system as a "complex of elements in mutual interaction"; Anatol Rapoport stated that a "whole which functions as a whole by virtue of the interdependence of its parts is called a system";[22] and R. L. Ackoff wrote that initially "we can define a system broadly and crudely as any entity, conceptual or physical, which consists of interdependent parts."[23] These definitions show that no significant advance in thinking about the generalized concept of a system has taken place since the late nineteenth century. The Haldane brothers and the biologist Edmund Montgomery, the organicists discussed earlier, in fact had ideas that ran parallel to those of mid-twentieth-century system theorists.

It is apparent that the same reasoning underlies these various cases: the principles that led Montgomery to identify the whole as being the individual biological organism also led the Haldanes and the Hegelians to their respective views. An exactly similar situation exists for general system theorists; and the concept of "system" with which they operate provides no ground for limiting their attention to anything but the universe as a whole. An example should make the point clear. Suppose a general system theorist is treating an army unit as a system. Now, if a system is a "complex of elements in interaction," it can be argued with some justice that an army unit is not an independent system, for it is itself interrelated with many other "entities" to form a larger system, the entire army. And once the theorist has embarked on this road—as in fact he does when he defines a system as "elements in interaction"—he seems committed to continuing his journey until he joins the Hegelians in contemplating the whole of reality!

This difficulty has been recognized by at least one system theorist. Stafford Beer, in a paper presented to the First Systems Symposium at Case Institute of Technology, stated: "Earlier it was contended that the boundaries of a system are subjective; and this is strongly supported at the philosophical level by the Hegelian axiom of internal relations—which of course makes it logically possible to equate every system with the universe itself. So the crucial scientific problem for systems research is this: how to separate a particular viable system for study from the rest of the universe without committing an annihilating *divisio*. . . . These are problems of desperate urgency for every nontrivial systems study."*

* Stafford Beer, "Below the Twilight Arch: A Mythology of Systems," in Eckman, pp. 18–19. A. D. Hall and R. E. Fagen, in a paper

Beer is not exaggerating when he calls this a problem of desperate urgency; and he is also right in raising the issue of triviality. It is indeed trivial to define a system in terms of the interrelation of components; for every entity in the universe enters into *some* relationships, and everything, therefore, can be regarded as a component in some sort of system.* The general system theorists' definition of a system, seen in this light, is not particularly informative. In effect, the definition tells us that a system is something composed of any things interrelated in any way. For sheer profundity, this bears comparison with William James's famous parody of the definition of evolution: "Evolution is a change from a no-howish untalkaboutable all-alikeness to a some-howish and in-general talkaboutable not-all-alikeness by continuous sticktogetherations and somethingelseifications."[24]

It might be thought that the system theorists' problem of specifying what they mean by a system has a simple solution. Why not simply select certain interrelated entities that happen to be of relevance to a particular investigation, and then call this group of entities a system?[25] But this cure turns out to be far worse than the original disease, for it runs afoul of some of the funda-

on systems engineering, raise the same problem in another form. They define the environment of a system as that which is in interrelation with the system, and this leads them to the problem of distinguishing when an object belongs to a system and when it belongs to the environment. "The answer is by no means definite." See Hall and Fagen, "Definition of System," in Buckley, *Modern Systems Research*, p. 83.

* Hall and Fagen (p. 82) acknowledge this: "For any given set of objects it is impossible to say that no interrelationships exist."

mental principles of GST. In the first place, the theorist can only select relevant entities if he has some principles of selection or criteria of relevance; and he can only have these for a particular problem if investigation has been under way and has already made considerable progress. He must have reached the stage where it is possible to say that entities *A*, *B*, and *C* are relevant and entities *D*, *E*, and *F* are not. Moreover, this fairly advanced stage of investigation must have been reached without using system methods, since what is required here is the information necessary *before* a system theorist can select or define his system. In fact, it is quite likely that the mechanistic or analytic method, which general system theorists claim is not applicable, has been the method used to achieve whatever important advances have been made in the investigation.

A second objection to the simple cure—selecting the entities that form a relevant system—is that the general system theorist has not gone far enough. He also has to show that in isolating this system from the other entities with which it is normally interrelated he has not introduced artifacts, or as Beer put it, that he has not committed an "annihilating *divisio*." One of the main points made by GST is that the interrelationships between parts of a system are of vital importance. And in isolating a system for study the theorist is necessarily severing some interrelationships—the very thing his own creed tells him should not be done.

3. *Vagueness over what is to be included within system theory.* In Bertalanffy's early explanation, GST had as

its subject matter "the formulation and derivation of those principles which hold for systems in general."[26] In subsequent years, however, a puzzling situation developed. Some works on GST have put forward *classifications* of systems,[27] whereas others have contained discussions of concepts important in investigations of systems—wholeness, sum, emergence, open and closed systems, the entropy of systems, the principle of equifinality, and so on.[28] But the most puzzling feature emerges clearly in a 1962 essay by Bertalanffy, which distinguishes between system theory in "the broad sense" and General System Theory "in the narrower sense." Bertalanffy identifies seven different bodies of theory as constituting system theory in "the broad sense": cybernetics, information theory, game theory, decision theory, topology, factor analysis, and finally GST.[29]

The puzzle here is what these seven areas of system theory have in common, apart from the trivial fact that the word "system" can be applied to all of them. Certainly GST is different in kind from the other six bodies of theory mentioned by Bertalanffy; and if these six are regarded as second-order studies, then GST is at an even greater level of abstraction and must be classified as a third-order study.* Thus it is a serious mistake to group

---

* According to the usage adopted here, a first-order study would be a study of "particulars"—e.g. a particular feedback system. A second-order study would be at the next level of generality—e.g. a study of feedback systems in general. And a third-order study would be even more general—e.g. a study of many different *types* of system (feedback, information, biological, and so on).

these seven studies together as though they were analogous or parallel.

Another point is that the opposition of GST to the mechanistic or analytic method, and its resemblances to Hegelianism and the biological organicism of the turn of the century, mark it as quite different from the other six areas of theory. If these basic tenets of GST were rejected, the other six bodies of theory identified by Bertalanffy would presumably stand virtually unshaken. Or to put the point another way, studies and theories on a lower order of abstraction are always able to survive the demise of a theory on a higher order; thus the six second-order system studies could survive the death of the third-order study, GST. The objections raised here against GST do not necessarily apply to these other areas of "system theory in the broad sense."

4. *The failure of GST as a scientific theory.* Perhaps the most important feature of a scientific theory is its value in predicting some future observable event. Karl Popper has explicated this function of science in detail, and has argued that nonscientific theories (or pseudoscientific theories) do not have predictive value.[30] It is interesting to consider GST in the light of Popper's remarks. Like Marxism or Freudianism (which Popper has attacked directly), GST is wise after the event. It is always possible for a general system theorist to explain in his own theoretical terms what has happened in a particular system he is investigating—*after* the "happening" has taken place. The system theorist's predictions

before an event are usually not predictions in the scientific sense at all, for they are far too vague. (The exception would be when the theorist is investigating systems where precise laws have been discovered by traditional mechanistic means—e.g. electronics circuits, mechanical systems, or certain physiological systems.)

As an example of the weakness of system theory with respect to predictive power, consider Philip H. Coombs's book *The World Educational Crisis: A Systems Analysis*. Under UNESCO sponsorship, Coombs studied the educational systems of many emerging and developed nations, his aim being to determine the effects on these systems of changes in various of their parts. He concentrated on such things as shortage of teachers, increases in costs, and increases in the number of pupils—all changes that have contributed to the present world crisis in education. It is a marked feature of Coombs's book that he is unable to make precise predictions. From the fact that a given educational system has had a threefold increase in incoming pupils in a very short period, for example, he cannot predict how the system will adjust to this serious alteration of input. It is a truism to say that some changes must occur; and it is possible to guess at the most likely changes, since the range of possibilities here is a fairly limited one. But in order to make this sort of speculative hypothesis one does not have to be a system theorist.

This weakness of GST seems to have been recognized even by its keenest supporter. Perhaps it is well to allow

Bertalanffy to have the final word: "The decisive question is that of the explanatory and predictive value of the 'new theories' attacking the host of problems around wholeness, teleology, etc. . . . There is no question that new horizons have been opened up, but the relations to empirical facts often remain tenuous."[31]

5

Systems, Holons, and Politics

I T IS NOT enough just to criticize system theory along the lines of Chapter 4. This approach highlights weaknesses at the expense of any strengths, and it obscures features of the theory that have made it so appealing. It will be easier to perceive some of these strengths, and, paradoxically, to realize how closely they are related to the weaknesses, in the context of some fairly detailed applications of system theory in the human sciences.

Arthur Koestler's trilogy including *The Sleepwalkers* and *The Act of Creation* was completed in 1967 with *The Ghost in the Machine*. In this last work, Bertalanffy received eleven citations in the index, and Paul Weiss four. Koestler himself was quite specific about the book's affiliations, for he wrote that part of the material of the book could be called "an exercise in 'general system theory.' "[1] For the convenience of his readers Koestler summarized the key points of his argument in an appendix entitled "General Properties of Open Hierarchical Systems." It is apparent from these pages that system theory was the unquestioned background for Koestler's work.

Having examined some of the glories of the human intellect—science and art—in his previous books, Koestler turned his attention to its "pathology." In the first hundred pages or so of *The Ghost in the Machine* he developed a theoretical framework in terms of which he argued the rest of his case, and it was in this opening section that the influence of system theory was most marked.

Koestler's general theme, illustrated by examples from many human sciences but particularly from biology and psychology, was that crude atomistic theories must now be replaced by a conception of hierarchical systems. Although the terminology was loose, his central thesis appears to have fallen under the ambit of Holism 3; in essence, he was advocating conceptual reform: "The concept of hierarchic order occupies a central place in this book, and lest the reader should think that I am riding a private hobby horse, let me reassure him that this concept has a long and respectable ancestry. So much so, that defenders of orthodoxy are inclined to dismiss it as 'old hat'—and often in the same breath to deny its validity. Yet I hope to show as we go along that this old hat, handled with some affection, can produce lively rabbits."[2] And as he added in a footnote, "The word 'hierarchy' does not even appear in the index of most modern textbooks of psychology or biology."

To facilitate his discussion of hierarchical systems,

Koestler coined the term "holon." A holon is "Janus-faced": seen from a point of view "below" it in the system, it is a self-contained whole; but from a vantage point "above" it in the hierarchy, it is a dependent part.[3] Koestler argued that wholes and parts in an absolute sense do not exist anywhere, either among living organisms or among social organizations. "What we find are intermediary structures on a series of levels in an ascending order of complexity: sub-wholes which display, according to the way you look at them, some of the characteristics commonly attributed to wholes and some of the characteristics commonly attributed to parts."[4]

Koestler's chief target, using this interesting notion, was behavioristic psychology, and in particular the model of human language as a complex chain of stimuli and responses. Far more credible, Koestler argued (drawing support from Noam Chomsky and others), was the treelike, multi-leveled, "hierarchically ordered systems" model of language.[5] Active speech, Koestler wrote, "consists in the stepwise elaboration, articulation, concretization, of originally inarticulate generalized intents. The branching of the tree symbolizes this step-by-step, hierarchic process of spelling out the implicit idea in explicit terms, of converting the potentialities of an idea into the actual motion-patterns of the vocal cords. The process has been compared to the development of the embryo: the fertilized egg contains all the potentialities of the future individual; these are then 'spelled out' in successive stages of differentiation."[6]

It is not necessary to see eye to eye with Koestler regarding his examples in order to appreciate the suggestiveness and explanatory usefulness of the conceptual enrichment that he was advocating. Moreover, as suggested earlier, one does not have to abandon the analytic method or reductionism in order to appreciate the value of such concepts as "hierarchy" and "holon." Science does grow, and has grown, as a result of conceptual enrichment of this kind, and there is no conflict between it and Holism 3. The issue here is central. Koestler saw a conflict because he regarded what he was advocating as more than conceptual reform: in his eyes, the acceptance of concepts like "holon" and "hierarchy" in the human sciences would be a methodological breakthrough. And he was able to hold this view because his analysis of the key ideas of "mechanism," "atomism," and "holism" was too crude, in that he did not distinguish between the quite different theses often lumped together under one or another of these labels. Thus he seemed to have few qualms when he stated that the "concept of the holon, and of the Open Hierarchic System, attempts to reconcile atomism and holism."[7] The oddity of claiming that two "concepts" could reconcile these "isms" escaped him.

The confusion in Koestler's notion of holism can be illustrated in terms of the very parable he used to introduce the concept of a holon, the story of the two watchmakers Bios and Mekhos.[8] Mekhos made his watches by piecing together the parts one by one; but Bios joined a small number of parts together into a subgroup, then put several of these together to form a larger grouping, and so on until the job was finished. Bios prospered, but Mekhos was forced out of business, the reason being that when interruptions came and Mekhos put down his partially completed watch it disintegrated into parts, whereas Bios's watch only broke down into subgroups, which were much easier to piece together. According to Koestler's calculation, Mekhos would take on the average several thousand times longer than Bios to complete one watch.

Koestler did not make clear exactly what it was that was shown by this parable. But clues can be obtained from the remainder of the chapter that began with this horological tale. In the first place, Koestler concluded that in the evolutionary development of life hierarchical development via stable subgroups, in the manner of Bios, must have played a key role; for only such a course would have allowed the present stage of evolutionary development to have been reached in the time available, and there would have been as an additional advantage the greater resistance to damage that Bios's method conferred.

Though the case for stable subgroups was reasonable, Koestler's argument was not conclusive in showing Bios to have an advantage over Mekhos here. Suppose the elementary units that eventually become connected are 1, 2, 3, 4, 5, ... 1,000. Bios takes 1 through 4 and joins these to form stable subgroup *A*. He makes another group, *B*, from 5–8, and *C* from 9–12. He thus continues working up to part 1,000, constructing subgroups, whereupon he starts to link these to form larger groups. During this time—for simplicity let us suppose it is when he is working with part 10—an interruption occurs. Bios is left with stable subgroups *A* and *B*, but group *C* (which he had not completed) will disintegrate. Here Mekhos is at no disadvantage at all. He starts by joining parts 1 and 2, then adds 3, 4, 5, and so on. When the interruption comes at part 10, Mekhos in effect will also be left with stable subgroups *A* and *B* (parts 1–4 and 5–8, respectively).

As an illustration of the deficiencies of the analytic method, the parable is even less effective. A number of different theoretical issues can be distinguished in the watchmaking analogy, and the story of Bios and Mekhos as told by Koestler does nothing to clarify these:

1. There is the matter of the initial design of the watch—is it theoretically possible to produce a time-piece?

2. What is the best method of actually carrying out the construction?

3. Could all the properties of the completed timepiece (e.g. precision, relative silence of the movement, or resistance to shock) be predicted *beforehand* from a knowledge of the parts only?

4. Could all the properties of the watch be explained *afterward* by reference to the properties of the parts?

5. Would it be useful to introduce new concepts into horological literature to facilitate technical discussions?

The first question raised is a technical one, and Koestler chooses to ignore it. Issue 2, though also technical, is the only one he actually tackles; and his somewhat questionable answer is that the method of Bios is superior, for watchmakers, to that of Mekhos. It is in items 3–5 that the issues of analysis, reductionism, and holism come to the fore, and these are what Koestler fails to discuss in his parable.

In 3, the supporter of organicism, or Holism 1, would be tempted to take the negative in opposition to an affirmative argued by supporters of the analytic method. ("Tempted" because, after all, the example is one of watchmaking—a case where organicists would usually concede the point. But anything can happen in a parable.) In 4, the supporter of Holism 2 would be tempted to take the negative in opposition to a reductionist or mechanist, who would argue that certainly all the properties of the whole, after they had been discovered, could be explained in terms of the properties of the parts. In 5, the supporter of Holism 3 might argue that terms such as "holon" foster useful discussion of the properties of groups and should be widely adopted. The analyst and reductionist might or might not agree with him, according to the strength of his argument; but Holism 3 is not incompatible with their positions.

To Koestler, who ignores the important distinction between the three types of holism, the whole matter is simple. As he put it a few pages after introducing the parable: "We can 'dissect' a complex whole into its composite holons of the second and third order, and so on, but we cannot 'reduce' it to a sum of its parts, nor predict its properties from those of its parts. The hierarchy concept of 'levels of organization' in itself implies a re-

jection of the reductionist view that all phenomena of
life (consciousness included) can be reduced to and explained by physico-chemical laws."⁹

The study of political life presents a few more problems
than watchmaking, and in confronting these system
theory has displayed its best features. In general, the field
of political analysis has been marred by a lack of agreement on terminology and on what concepts best aid the
formation of explanatory theories. In recent years David
Easton has argued that system theory can provide a
unifying framework within which theorists can proceed toward the development of a body of "empirical
theory."¹⁰

In *A Systems Analysis of Political Life* (1965) Easton
argues in some detail that it is fruitful to treat the political system—any political system—as an open system
having inputs, interactions, outputs, and feedback loops.
He identifies the major types of each of these processes
in a way that other political scientists have found very
helpful. As one reviewer put it, "The detailed concepts
in *A Systems Analysis of Political Life* will help illumi-
nate inquiry into *any* of the traditional fields of special-
ization.... They have already been—and will increasingly be—of great value to careful fact gatherers, narrow-
gauge theorists and broader-gauge theorists. The book
has already become, in my judgment, 'must reading.' "¹¹
In light of this, it is interesting to inquire further into
Easton's conception of system theory.

It is clear from an examination of Easton's books that

he finds the model of political life as a system with inputs and so on to be fruitful, but equally clear that he has abandoned some central features of system theory that set it in opposition to the analytic method. In other words, Easton appears to have adopted a system approach because it provides a convenient framework and is a fruitful model; he does not adopt it because of its holistic features, and in fact it is these that he either specifically rejects or simply refuses to make use of.

Something of Easton's attitude emerges when he writes: "No one way of conceptualizing any major area of human behavior will do full justice to all its variety and complexity. Each type of theoretical orientation brings to the surface a different set of problems, provides unique insights and emphases, and thereby makes it possible for alternative and even competing theories to be equally and simultaneously useful, although often for quite different purposes. The conceptual orientation that I am proposing—systems analysis—is one that stems from the fundamental decision to view political life as a system of behavior."[12]

Easton's refusal to accept the holistic aspects of system theory becomes manifest in his discussion of how a system can usefully be selected for study from among all the interrelated parts of nature. This, it will be recalled, was the problem that Stafford Beer identified as having "desperate urgency for every nontrivial systems study"— "how to separate a particular viable system for study from the rest of the universe without committing an annihilating *divisio*."[13]

Easton considers two opposed solutions. First, "whether or not a set of interactions constitutes a system will depend upon the extent to which they naturally cohere. From this point of view, systems are given in nature." Second, "all systems are constructs of the mind. We might maintain that it is pointless to try to distinguish so-called natural from nonnatural or nonexistent systems. In this interpretation any aggregate of interactions that we choose to identify may be said to form a system."[14] Of these two alternatives, supporters of Holism 1 must take the first. Just any part of nature cannot be taken and called a system, for this could sever vital interrelationships; the resulting object of study would be an artifact, not a system wherein the whole was more than the sum of the parts. But Easton opts for the second alternative, and thus is breaking with holism.

Easton cites three arguments in support of his choice. First, even if systems were to be regarded as naturally occurring entities, one would be no further toward solving the practical problem of actually locating such systems. An investigator could not be sure that what had been called a natural system was indeed a system until after he had done further work and "gone through the motions." Second, Easton argues, there is little problem in distinguishing a natural system when its components are "tightly connected."* But of course a natural system can easily have "loosely associated" components,

---

* The second and third arguments are directed, in effect, at the weakness of system theorists' definition of a system as "elements in interaction" (a weakness pointed out in Chapter 4).

with the result that "a considerable change in one has negligible or no discernible effects on the other." In such cases, where is the line to be drawn between members and nonmembers of the system? At what point will the components be regarded as a random collection rather than a natural system? Third, Easton points out that not all covariance between components would "intuitively meet the criteria of a system." Often, two entities appear to be related, but no explanation of the relation can yet be offered. Until one is forthcoming, it is questionable whether the entities form a system; at the very least, evidence is required "to demonstrate the genuineness of the interdependence."[15]

It is apparent from Easton's discussion that he does not regard the relationships between the components of the political systems he is analyzing as being organic or internal. In one revealing passage he tackles the question that all neo-Hegelians eventually had to face: "What is there to prevent us from stating that everything in the world is related to everything else, thereby combining all social life into one grand system?" His answer is most un-Hegelian: "Although there is no logical reason why this could not be done, it is more significant to point out that there is no positive reason for doing so."[16] To write this way is to depart from the arguments of the founders of GST.

Though not an organicist, then, Easton has been extremely sensitive to the need to take interrelationships into account in the human sciences: "It is commonplace in political research to say that at one level of analysis, everything seems to be related to everything else. And even though typically we must chop off a segment of reality for specific research, it is always with the knowledge that somehow we are violating reality. For empirical purposes this is unavoidable and does little damage as long as we are sharply aware of what we are about. But from a theoretical point of view, it is crucial that we devise a set of perspectives and parallel categories that permit us to formulate the basic analytic questions in such a way as to take the interrelationship of political phenomena into account, and not in any trivial sense."[17] There is much to commend and little to condemn in this passage. To do the things discussed here, without recourse to Holism 1 or Holism 2, is certainly not objectionable.

6

Structure and Function

No doubt largely owing to the pervasive influence of Darwinism, the biology, sociology, and anthropology of the second half of the nineteenth century typically held structure and function to be two sides of one coin. Herbert Spencer, for example, regarded both organisms and societies as having structures—systems for circulating nutriment, centers of command, and so on—which performed functions having survival value. The conception was relatively straightforward, and the logic was easy to comprehend.

In the twentieth century, however, the concepts of structure and function have taken on a complexity, and a Hegelian logic, that makes them far from straightforward. One has only to look at the maze that many writers create in their efforts to define what, in current literature, is meant by these terms. As one authority puts it, the usage of the term "structure" provokes "a degree of pleasant puzzlement"; and the same could be said of "function." One of the few undeniable statements that can be made about the two terms in contemporary hu-

man science is that both of them often have holistic con-
notations.

It does not seem possible to express the essence of contemporary structuralism in an elegant definition. Jonathan Culler's recent judgment seems appropriate
(though he himself has considered it somewhat harsh):
"Structure, we are repeatedly told, is not an abstract form
but content itself, grasped in its logical organization;
but seldom is this article of faith more blatantly flouted
than in general discussions of structuralism, where the
relations of part and whole ... often fail to materialize
in the articles themselves.... The observers often feel
that despite the elegance of the proceedings no common
quarry has been flushed. They depart with nothing—no
common method or theory—that they can point to and
call 'structuralism.' It may be, of course, that the term
has outlived its usefulness. To call oneself a structuralist
was always a polemical gesture, a way of attracting attention and associating oneself with others whose work
was of moment; and, therefore, by the time structuralism became the subject of colloquia it had taken so many
guises that little could be gained from using the term."[1]

Nevertheless, it is possible to find a basic thesis common to much structuralist writing: namely, that all human social phenomena are structured rather than random. The problem is that this structure is deep-seated
and is not apparent on cursory inspection. As Claude
Lévi-Strauss puts it: "If, as we believe to be the case, the
unconscious activity of the mind consists in imposing

forms upon content, and if these forms are fundamentally the same for all minds—ancient and modern, primitive and civilized (as the study of the symbolic function, expressed in language, so strikingly indicates)—it is necessary and sufficient to grasp the unconscious structure underlying each institution and each custom, in order to obtain a principle of interpretation valid for other institutions and other customs, provided of course that the analysis is carried far enough."[2]

But by itself this is not "necessary and sufficient" to make structuralism comprehensible. Men use the things about them—clothing, food, natural objects—not only in ways that reflect their biological needs for food, shelter, and security, but also in ways that reflect social rules, social meanings, and so on. The social meanings given to clothing, to food, to the way we talk to each other and treat each other, or to our myths and legends are not random; indeed, these manifestations of human social activity can be regarded as languages, in the formal sense of the term.[3] It is here that underlying patterns or structures can be detected.

However, the analysis must go deep; the structure will not be discovered if it is only the signs or elements that are examined—the clothing, the food, the stories, and so on. The structure only becomes evident when the *relations* between elements are considered. And hence—the argument runs—a system view must be adopted, and the whole set of relations between elements must be studied in order to ascertain the relations between these relations: "It is the *relations* between the elements and

not the elements themselves which are significant. . . .
This is the basis of Lévi-Strauss' 'transformational method.' According to this method, when one is considering
a group of myths, for example, the problem is not to find
inductive generalizations which are true of them or of
their elements, but to consider each as a transform of the
other, a variant in which change of elements accom-
panies a preservation of relations, or of relations of relations. . . . That structure is not of the order of observable
fact is one of Lévi-Strauss' persistent themes."[4] It is in
this involved context that the structuralists make their
various holistic claims.

In expounding structuralism in general, Lévi-Strauss,
Jean Piaget, and other scholars have acknowledged a
considerable debt to the field of linguistics. Lévi-Strauss
noted approvingly one "programmatic statement" by N.
Troubetzkoy, "the illustrious founder of structural linguistics," in which the structural method was reduced
to four basic operations: "First, structural linguistics
shifts from the study of *conscious* linguistic phenomena
to study of their *unconscious* infrastructure; second, it
does not treat *terms* as independent entities, taking instead as its basis of analysis the *relations* between terms;
third, it introduces the concept of *system*—'modern
phonemics does not merely proclaim that phonemes are
always part of a system; it *shows* concrete phonemic
systems and elucidates their structure'; finally, structural
linguistics aims at discovering *general laws*, either by in-
duction 'or . . . by logical deduction, which would give
them an absolute character.' "[5]

Piaget also acknowledged the debt to linguistics, and offered his own programmatic statement: "As a first approximation, we may say that a structure is a system of transformations. Inasmuch as it is a system and not a mere collection of elements and their properties, these transformations involve laws: the structure is preserved or enriched by the interplay of its transformation laws, which never yield results external to the system nor employ elements that are external to it. In short, the notion of structure is composed of three key ideas: the idea of wholeness, the idea of transformation, and the idea of self-regulation."[6]

The references in these two passages to systems, to relations, to wholeness, and to self-regulation raise the possibility that the whole gamut of holisms is in some way bound up with structuralism. Another example to focus the discussion, and one that is as clear—or as obscure—as any in structuralist literature, is Lévi-Strauss's handling of kinship, in particular the "problem of the avunculate." He distinguishes "two quite different orders of reality" in what is usually referred to as a kinship system: there are the terms used to express the various family relationships; and accompanying these is a "system of attitudes" such as respect, affection, and hostility.[7] The terminology will differ from culture to culture, and so may attitudes toward any given relative. In particular, there is an interesting variation across cultures in attitudes toward the mother's brother; and making sense of these permutations is the "problem of the avunculate."

Earlier writers had tended to regard the importance of

the mother's brother in certain societies simply as the survival of a previous system of matrilineal descent;[8] but the work of Lowie, and more particularly of Radcliffe-Brown, was revolutionary. Radcliffe-Brown noted that two "antithetical systems of attitudes" were involved. In some societies the maternal uncle represented family authority, whereas in others he was on very familiar terms with his nephew. Additionally, there seemed to be an inverse relationship between a boy's attitude toward his father and his attitude toward his maternal uncle: in cases where he was very familiar toward one, he was invariably respectful toward the other. Radcliffe-Brown concluded that in patrilineal societies it was the father who was the authority figure, and that in matrilineal societies it was the maternal uncle.[9]

Lévi-Strauss's structuralism comes to the fore in his rejection of Radcliffe-Brown's work: "We should certainly recognize that Radcliffe-Brown's article leaves unanswered some fundamental questions. First, the avunculate does not occur in all matrilineal or all patrilineal systems, and we find it present in some systems which are neither matrilineal nor patrilineal. Further, the avuncular relationship is not limited to two terms, but presupposes four, namely, brother, sister, brother-in-law, and nephew. An interpretation such as Radcliffe-Brown's arbitrarily isolates particular elements of a global structure which must be treated as a whole."[10]

Looking at more societies, Lévi-Strauss felt able to identify the whole system of which Radcliffe-Brown had studied only a part, and to formulate the underlying structural law: "When we consider societies of the Cherkness and Trobriand types it is not enough to study the correlation of attitudes between *father/son* and *uncle/sister's son*. This correlation is only one aspect of a global system containing four types of relationships which are organically linked, namely: *brother/sister, husband/wife, father/son,* and *mother's brother/sister's son*. The two groups in our example illustrate a law which can be formulated as follows: In both groups, the relation between maternal uncle and nephew is to the relation between brother and sister as the relation between father and son is to that between husband and wife. Thus if we know one pair of relations, it is always possible to infer the other."[11]

It is now possible to answer the question raised earlier: what holistic theses are present in structuralism? In the first place, Lévi-Strauss's remarks seem to lend support to the structuralist Raymond Boudon, who related the rise of structuralism to the abandonment of Galileo's "simple-minded epistemology," according to which science should remain "the field of mechanistic explanations."[12] In this view, structuralism was close to Holism 1. Lévi-Strauss suggested that Radcliffe-Brown was an adherent of mechanism and atomism, and the further charge that the latter had isolated "particular elements of a global structure" seems to reflect Lévi-Strauss's own adherence to the basic ideas of the organismic archetype, Holism 1. But of what was Radcliffe-Brown guilty? According to the passage cited a little earlier, he had tried to solve the problem of the avunculate in terms of relations between father, son, and maternal uncle; Lévi-Strauss claimed that this approach isolated one part from the whole global system composed of brother, sister, husband, wife, father, son, maternal uncle, and nephew.

But Lévi-Strauss was mistaken in thinking that he had here established the worth of a systems or antimechanistic approach. In fact, he had not established that elements of the kinship system change their essential properties when isolated from the whole of which they are supposed to be parts (Holism 1). Nor had he shown that the whole system cannot be explained in terms of the behavior of the parts (Holism 2). What he was saying, in effect, was not in conflict with mechanism and reductionism at all: Radcliffe-Brown simply had not taken enough variables into account. Many mechanistic theories of the past were faulty not because of some defect in mechanism, but because the science—the information-gathering—simply was not adequate. If Lévi-Strauss is to be believed, Radcliffe-Brown's theory falls into this category; his solution to the problem of the avunculate was oversimplified and did not account for all the facts.

Lévi-Strauss himself was doing something commonplace in traditional science: that is, offering a more complex theory based on the study of a greater number of variables. Moreover, it is virtually certain that the method of investigation that led to this theory was analytic (i.e. piecemeal) rather than holistic. Lévi-Strauss collated data concerning the degree of familiarity or respect in relationships such as those between father and son or sister and brother—a typical analytic procedure. He studied not the whole as such, but rather the relationships between various pairs of parts (more parts, of course, than had been studied by Radcliffe-Brown).

Lévi-Strauss, then, was considerably overstating his case when he summarized the main part of his discussion: "Thus we see that in order to understand the avunculate we must treat it as one relationship within a system, while the system itself must be considered as a whole in order to grasp its structure. This structure rests upon four terms (brother, sister, father, and son), which are linked by two pairs of correlative oppositions in such a way that in each of the two generations there is always a positive relationship and a negative one."[13]

A further element of holism in the structuralist position is connected with the distinction between the synchronic and the diachronic. Lévi-Strauss explained this distinction using the example of an orchestral score: music can be read diachronically, from left to right, or synchronically, along the vertical axis.[14] In other words, a diachronic study is the study of successive states, such as the development of a musical theme; a synchronic study concerns the interrelationships that exist at any one time, such as those between the instruments of the orchestra playing in harmony. It is the synchronic form of study that structuralists view as the core of linguistics and anthropology. As Piaget notes, "structuralism is chiefly a departure from the diachronic study of isolated linguistic phenomena which prevailed in the nineteenth century and a turn to the investigation of synchronously functioning unified language systems."[15]

The synchronic/diachronic distinction, and a concomitant emphasis on synchronic study, are common in holist literature, although the ideas are often expressed in different terminology. In particular, this approach has been prominent in the writings of those who have wedded holism to functionalism; and it will be useful to examine this aspect of the matter before proceeding.

Although in some respects functionalism, like organicism and system theory, can be traced back to the ancient world, its modern life dates from the mid-nineteenth century. As Horace Kallen notes in the *Encyclopedia of the Social Sciences*, "Functionalism is a term which came into the foreground of philosophic discourse in the last quarter of the nineteenth century and has maintained an increasingly strong position there ever since. It sums up and designates the most general of the many consequences of the impact of Darwinism upon the sciences of man and nature."[16]
It is true that several of the founders of modern functionalism were evolutionists—Herbert Spencer in sociology and John Dewey in psychology and philosophy stand out—but to admit this is not to acknowledge that an evolutionary framework is a necessary part of functionalism. And to talk of functionalism is not to concede that the term is used in only one sense in the social sciences; indeed, a brief survey of the literature reveals much terminological confusion. Rather than stipulating a definition here, it seems better to illustrate one common usage of the term by considering a case history.

One of the main directions in which Darwin's work was to influence thought outside biology had already been indicated before the publication of *Origin of Species* in 1859; for Herbert Spencer, the "apostle of selfhelp," had been applying evolutionary ideas to a wide range of topics since the beginning of the 1850's.[17] Spencer had met evolutionary theory in its pre-Darwinian form even earlier, when he developed an interest in geology while working as a railway construction engineer in 1840. He purchased Lyell's *Principles of Geology*, and in it found a refutation of the evolutionary views put forward by the Chevalier de Lamarck. With a certain natural perversity, he instantly adopted Lamarck's most notorious thesis— the inheritance of acquired characteristics—and during the next few years he maintained his interest by reading a number of works touching on the subject. In the course of writing a book review in 1851 he came across the other key to what was to become his lifelong world view. This was the work of the embryologist Karl von Baer, who had suggested that all embryonic development follows a path of increasing complexity—that homogeneity of structure is always replaced by heterogeneity.[18]

These two principles merged together in Spencer's mind, and he came to think of evolutionary advance in terms of an increasing complexity of structure. In his early essay "Progress: Its Law and Cause" (1857), he wrote: "From the remotest past which Science can fathom, up to the novelties of yesterday, that in which Progress essentially consists is the transformation of the homogeneous into the heterogeneous."[19] Later he developed the same idea into his famous law: "Evolution is an integration of matter and concomitant dissipation of motion; during which the matter passes from an indefinite, incoherent homogeneity to a definite, coherent heterogeneity; and during which the retained motion undergoes a parallel transformation."[20] The mechanistic bent of Spencer's mind was displayed in his further argument that the transformation of the homogeneous was an inevitable result of each physical cause having more than one effect.

This form of evolutionism was a rich source of confusion and obscurity. It led Spencer to treat the growth of an individual and the evolution of a species as similar processes; and he subsumed both, together with such things as stellar evolution and the development of societies, in the "increase in heterogeneity" formula. But buried here, too, was the seed of his functionalism. This can be seen in *Principles of Sociology* (1876), where he wrote: "In societies, as in living bodies, increase of mass is habitually accompanied by increase of structure. Along with that integration which is the primary trait of evolution, both exhibit in high degrees the secondary trait, differentiation."[21] Later in the same work Spencer pointed out that "changes of structures cannot occur without changes of function."[22] In fact, he had found it impossible earlier in the book to discuss changes in structure without referring to the parallel changes in function.

Keeping close to a path he had blazed earlier (in "The Social Organism," 1863), Spencer argued that a society and an organism had many functional needs in common.

Both had to distribute nutriment to individual members, both needed a center of government and channels of communication, and so on. He was so excited by these parallels that at times he seemed to be suggesting that the argument was not merely an analogy, and that a society actually *was* a single organism.

The extent to which functionalism was entangled with Spencer's ideas about evolution, growth, embryonic development, and society as an organism is illustrated by his treatment of the function and rise of chieftains in primitive society. The discussion opens with a reference to his own *Principles of Biology*, in which he claimed to have established "the general law that large aggregates have high organizations." Spencer had no qualms about applying this generalization to societies: "The social aggregate, homogeneous when minute, habitually gains in heterogeneity along with each increment of growth." Thus he saw groups of Eskimos, Australian aborigines, Bushmen, and Fuegians as being so homogeneous that they did not even have a "settled chieftainship." The members of these groups were similar in capability, and each could perform all the tasks necessary for survival. But when these "incoherent" and "headless" clusters reached the size of about one hundred members the function of maintenance necessitated the development of "a simple or compound ruling agency." This evolution of chieftainship was generally followed by a functional division of the group to foster regulative and operative activities, the men working in one sphere and the women in another.[23]

The growth and developing organization of a tribe, with a concomitant increase in efficiency, could lead to the capturing of slaves and the eventual amalgamation of the tribe with similar groups. "The holding together of the compound cluster implies a head of the whole as well as heads of the parts; and a differentiation analogous to that which originally produced a chief now produces a chief of chiefs. Sometimes the combination is made for defence against a common foe, and sometimes it results from conquest by one tribe of the rest."[24] Moreover, the union of various groups could facilitate the exchange of commodities between regions, and the groups might begin to specialize in certain types of products.

In summary, Spencer wrote: "The advance of organization which thus follows the advance of aggregation, alike in individual organisms and in social organisms, conforms in both cases to the same general law."[25] After restating his evolutionary law in simplified language, Spencer went on to illustrate it with the detailed example of the embryonic development of the vertebrate spinal column, nicely rounding off his mixture of incompatible ingredients.

A number of issues relevant to contemporary functionalism can be illustrated by reference to Spencer's work. One objection often advanced by twentieth-century opponents of the doctrine is that functionalism uses teleological explanations. Whereas scientists have traditionally explained the present and predicted the future on the basis of causes operating earlier in time, teleologists explain events in the present and the past in terms of causes

—purposes, ends, or final causes—that are located in the future. Thus Spencer was teleological when he wrote that sometimes primitive groups combine to face a common foe, for he was explaining a present or past phenomenon in terms of a future purpose or function.

One main objection to teleological explanation, in Carl Hempel's words, is that "in its more traditional forms, it fails to meet the minimum scientific requirement of empirical testability."[26] In other words, it is not clear what observations could confirm or refute such an explanation. However, Hempel is not completely hostile: "The functionalist mode of approach has proved illuminating, suggestive, and fruitful in many contexts. If the advantages it has to offer are to be reaped in full, it seems desirable and indeed necessary to pursue the investigation of specific functional relationships to the point where they can be expressed in terms of reasonably precise and objectively testable hypotheses."[27] In line with this view, Hempel feels that although functional explanations may seem particularly appropriate when a self-regulating or feedback system is being studied, it is always possible to rephrase them "in a more obviously causal form."[28]

Other writers have not been so moderate. Alan Ryan, referring to Hempel's "mistakes" regarding functionalism and teleology, asserts: "Teleological explanation . . . is necessarily holistic and causal, and is not—in spite of the claim of current orthodoxies—reducible in principle to explanation by mechanical causation."[29] Ryan is particularly impressed by the effectiveness of teleology in explaining self-regulating systems, but he still denies that society falls in this category, and hence is skeptical of functional explanations in discussions of social life.

By contrast, William Catton regards functionalism as having inherent dangers. He portrays sociology as developing from a prescientific animistic stage to one of scientific naturalism. However: "By adopting a functional approach we expose ourselves to special temptations to revert to animism, and special precautions become necessary if the benefits of naturalism are to be retained."[30]

Not all functional explanations are teleological, as Spencer's example of tribal alliance is. What is to be made of the same author's account of the rise of chieftains? Here Spencer pointed out the functional requirements of primitive groups with about one hundred members; and in explaining the origin of chieftains as a response to these requirements he was explaining the phenomenon in terms of prior causes, namely, the preexisting functional needs. This procedure would seem to avoid the charge of teleology.

Although Hempel and Catton both note that many functional explanations can be shown to be traditional causal or mechanistic explanations in disguise, they also emphasize the important minimum conditions that these explanations must satisfy. In brief, the possession of item i by a system s at time t can only be explained on the grounds that i satisfies functional need n of the system, provided this explanation is put forward in the context of a theory that determines what is meant by the expression "the functional needs of the system *s*." It would not be particularly convincing to explain that space monsters periodically visit Earth and eat large slabs of concrete because they have a functional need for it if we had no theory at all about the biology of space monsters. A functional explanation in such a context would merely be a cover for ignorance, much as when one of Molière's characters explains that opium puts people to sleep because of its "dormative power." However, if detailed information about the biochemistry of space monsters was available, and if it was revealed that one of their life-sustaining digestive enzymes required chemicals found in concrete, then we would be in a position to start offering functional explanations of their dietary habits.

But there is at least one other hurdle to cross. The functional need *n* having been established, in the context of a theory about the mechanisms involved in system *s*, it would still be necessary to show that the eating of concrete (*i*) is the only (or the most economical or pleasant) way to satisfy this need. As Hempel puts it: "It might well be that the occurrence of any one of a number of alternative items would suffice no less than the occurrence of *i* to satisfy requirement *n*, in which case the account provided ... simply fails to explain why the trait *i* rather than one of its alternatives is present in *s* at *t*."[31]

In the light of this discussion, Spencer's explanation that chieftains arose as a result of the functional requirements of primitive society is acceptable on formal grounds only if it satisfies these two minimal conditions: it must have been put forward in the context of a theory that defines these functional needs; and it must have been possible to establish that the rise of chieftains was the *only* way to satisfy some of these needs. It is here that the link between Spencer's functionalism and his eclectic evolutionary-embryological-social theories appears. In Spencer's view, social groups and individual organisms can be treated as obeying the same fundamental laws, so that there is a close parallel between the functional needs of organisms and social groups. In this context, his account of the development of leaders in primitive society is meaningful (although few today would accept either this account or Spencer's hodgepodge of biological and social theory). This does not mean that Spencer's explanation of the rise of chieftains is even formally valid, however, for he does not satisfy the second requirement by showing that there were no other possible ways to meet the social need.

Functional explanations put forward in disciplines other than sociology and biology must of course satisfy the same conditions. Consider the functional view of mind, or intellect, that was developed under the stimulus of Darwinian naturalism by William James, George H. Mead, John Dewey, and James R. Angell. According to evolutionary theory, species of organisms successful in the struggle for existence will possess adaptive features that confer some practical advantage—the capacity to hibernate or migrate during severe winters, the ability to make use of food sources not tapped by others, fleetness of foot, great strength, camouflage, the ability to maintain body temperature at a constant level in extreme environments, and so on.

The capacity for conscious thought can be viewed in this way as an adaptive feature functioning to confer an advantage in the struggle for existence. As William James put it: "Man, we now have reason to believe, has been evolved from infra-human ancestors, in whom pure reason hardly existed, if at all, and whose mind, so far as it can have had any function, would appear to have been an organ for adapting their movements to the impressions received from the environment, so as to escape the better from destruction. Consciousness would thus seem in the first instance to be nothing but a sort of superadded biological perfection—useless unless it prompted to useful conduct, and inexplicable apart from that consideration. . . . Man, whatever else he may be, is primarily a practical being, whose mind is given him to aid in adapting him to this world's life."[32]

This view, then, accounts for the capacity for conscious thought, i, of the species homo sapiens, s, in terms of satisfying the functional needs of survival and adaptation to the environment, n. It is clear that this view was put forward in the context of evolutionary theory, which specifies in general terms the meaning of the expression "functional needs of a species"; hence one of the two formal requirements for a valid functional explanation has been satisfied. The other requirement is that i must be shown to be the only, or the most efficacious, way of satisfying *n*. It is likely that this requirement could also be met; for the anthropoid apes from whom man evolved were creatures with only a few promising lines for future evolutionary development, and the capacity for thought was one of these.

Further clarification of the logic of all forms of functionalism has been provided by the sociologist Robert Merton, who points out that in the past many functional explanations confused functions that are "intended and recognized by participants" in the system under investigation with functions that are neither intended nor recognized.[33] Merton calls these manifest and latent functions, respectively. For example, the manifest function of a tribal rain dance is the production of rain—a function that it does not demonstrably fulfill—whereas the latent function of the ceremonial is the reinforcement of group identity.

Merton goes on to argue that a sociologist has much to gain, in terms of advancing his discipline, from concentrating on both types of function rather than focusing chiefly on manifest functions, as was usual in the past. Merton's discussion is wise, too, in avoiding a dangerous possibility opened up by his distinction, namely, the possibility of arguing that *all* facets of any system are functional (or dysfunctional), even if the participants in that system do not see them as such. "This universal functionalism may or may not be a heuristic postulate; that remains to be seen. But one should be prepared to find that it, too, diverts critical attention from a range of nonfunctional consequences of existing cultural forms."[34]

The examples of functionalism cited so far have all involved the theory of evolution in some way. A number of commentators would not regard this as accidental, for they see the two as being closely related. Horace Kallen, for example, states that functionalism "sums up and designates the most general of the many consequences of the impact of Darwinism."[35] And William Catton writes: "The tendency of functionalist literature to sound as if events are being explained in terms of final causes stems from neglect by the functionalists of the connection between functional analysis and evolutionary processes."[36]

The connection between functionalism and evolution, however, is not a necessary one. Functional explanations are only acceptable in the context of a theory that outlines the functional needs of a particular system; evolutionary theory can fill this role, but it is not the only theory that can do so. It is here that holism enters the picture. It is possible to discuss the operation of a complex entity not only in evolutionary terms but also in terms derived from organismic system theory—input, output, negative or positive feedback, and so on. Supporting this general analysis, several writers have noted that functionalism often appears in conjunction with organicism. Alan Ryan's statement is typical: "To be impressed by functionalist claims it is probably necessary to be impressed by the apparently organic nature of social life, and this means to be impressed by a seeming wisdom in the whole that does not stem from any of its members singly."[37]

There is some justification for this position. The central orientation of functionalism has been, in Merton's words, "the practice of interpreting data by establishing their consequences for larger structures in which they are implicated."[38] That is, item *i* is viewed in the light of its contribution toward meeting the requirements *n* of the system *s* in which it occurs. This analysis has sometimes been taken to indicate that the functionalist is logically committed to a type of system approach, in which *s* is an integrated whole whose parts (including *i*) contribute to its existence.

But this conclusion is unwarranted. A part can make important contributions to a system without the system being a whole or a unit in the organismic sense of Holism 1. Many nonorganismic wholes, in fact, have parts that contribute to their functioning in important ways. A clock, for example, is a mechanical aggregate of parts, each with its functional role; but the clockmaker who acknowledges this is not thereby committed to the view that his timepiece is an organismic system. Merton was possibly making a related point when he argued, "The assumption of the complete functional unity of human society is repeatedly contrary to fact."[39] In sum, it cannot be maintained that there is a *necessary* link between functionalism and organicism.

An example of functionalism that is at bottom neither evolutionary nor organismic (though it may have been influenced by both doctrines) is provided by the work of Sigmund Freud. His well-known structural division of the mind into id, ego, and superego, together with his account of their operation and the relationships between them, formed a framework in the context of which it was acceptable to offer functional explanations. After a series of consultations with a neurotic patient, for example, Freud might have concluded that the source of the trouble lay back in the patient's childhood, when he had felt a strong sexual attraction to his godmother, a desire that had subsequently been suppressed from consciousness and had only been revealed after painstaking psychoanalytic sessions. Why did suppression occur in this type of case?

Freud's explanation was both functional and teleological: "Even in organisms which later develop an efficient ego-organization, their ego is feeble and little differentiated from their id to begin with, during their first years of childhood. Imagine now what will happen if this powerless ego experiences an instinctual demand from the id which it would already like to resist (because it senses that to satisfy it is dangerous and would conjure up a traumatic situation, a collision with the external world) but which it cannot control.... In such a case the ego treats the instinctual danger as if it was an external one; it makes an attempt at flight, draws back from this portion of the id, and leaves it to its fate, after withholding from it all the contributions which it usually makes to instinctual impulses. The ego, as we put it, institutes a *repression* of these instinctual impulses. For the moment this has the effect of fending off the danger."[40]

In short, repression i is accounted for in terms of the functional need for protection from danger n of ego s.

It is not, then, a logical requirement that functionalism be linked with evolutionary theory or with organicism. Throughout its history, however, it has in fact often been linked with one or both of these, which has sometimes led to serious confusion.

In his attempt to account for the rise of chieftains in primitive society, Herbert Spencer oscillated between two methodological poles that he did not recognize as distinct. On one hand, he was interested in the evolutionary train of events, and he put forward genetic explanations to show that certain states of society led to others in which there was an increase in heterogeneity. But on the other hand, somewhat like the system analysts, he was interested in the actual functioning of a society at particular stages of its development and in relation to specific environments. Spencer was blind to the differences between these two approaches because he was under the illusion that his evolutionary law was applicable to *all* processes; he was disposed to unify and generalize, rather than to make distinctions and hence to increase complexity. His contemporary T. H. Huxley remarked with some justice that Spencer's idea of a tragedy was a theory killed by a fact.

John Stuart Mill saw somewhat more clearly the nature of the two modes of inquiry. He recognized what could be called a "horizontal" or functional mode that involved the relationships between coexisting parts of a society or other system at a given time; but he also discerned a "vertical" (genetic or historical) form of inquiry into the relationships between successive temporal stages of a system. Which type of inquiry was the fundamental one? "The uniformities of co-existence obtaining among phenomena which are effects of causes must (as we have so often observed) be corollaries from the laws of causation by which these phenomena are really determined. The mutual correlation between the different elements of each state of society is, therefore, a derivative law, resulting from the laws which regulate the succession between one state of society and another, for the proximate cause of every state of society is the state of society immediately preceding it. The fundamental problem, therefore, of the social science is to find the laws according to which any state of society produces the state which succeeds it and takes its place."[41]

The belief of both Mill and Spencer in the existence of laws determining the course of history is one that has not been shared by all subsequent investigators. Karl Popper has labeled it "historicism." In Popper's view, the study of history is "characterized by its interest in actual, singular, or specific events," and it is a serious mistake to believe that trains of events in nature proceed according to any given law or finite set of laws.[42] Each event is caused, but this does not mean that the train of events itself is subject to law. Popper cites the example of wind shaking a tree, whereupon Newton's apple falls to the ground. Involved in various parts of this simple chain of events are the laws of moving air, the laws of mechanics applicable to the flexibility of the tree branch, the law of gravitation, the laws of biochemistry relevant to the subsequent bruising of the apple, and so on; but there is no law determining the whole course of the sequence.[43]

Distinctions like that drawn by Mill between vertical and horizontal modes of inquiry are common in twentieth-century scholarship. It has already been remarked that structuralists distinguish in a similar way between the synchronic and the diachronic, and in the words of Piaget, "anthropological structuralism is, accordingly, firmly synchronic."[44] (Piaget himself, because of his interest in genetic or developmental processes, has a predilection for the diachronic approach.)

Earlier in the century, the social anthropologist A. R. Radcliffe-Brown clearly recognized that the genetic, evolutionary, or historical approach (the diachronic) was quite distinct from what he called the inductive or functional one (the synchronic). In his own field, he called the first approach ethnology and the second social anthropology. Ethnology suffered from the weakness that many of its "hypothetical reconstructions" of the course of past events could not be verified. In addition, historical and evolutionary investigations were based on assumptions that could not be established by ethnology—"assumptions as to the nature of culture and the laws of its development."[45]

It is central to Radcliffe-Brown's position that such laws can only be established by the functional (or inductive) investigations of social anthropology: "The functional method of interpretation rests on the assumption that a culture is an integrated system. In the life of a given community each element of the culture plays a specific part, has a specific function. The discovery of those functions is the task of a science that might be called 'social physiology'.... History, in the narrow sense, does not and cannot give us general laws. The hypothetical reconstruction of the past inevitably assumes certain general principles but does not prove them; on the contrary its results depend on their validity. The functional method aims at the discovery and verification of general laws by the same logical methods as those in use in the natural sciences—physics, chemistry, physiology."[46]

In effect, Radcliffe-Brown is distinguishing between the vertical level of genetic and historical inquiry and the more basic horizontal one of functional and inductive inquiry. Drawing the same distinction in a different terminology, Lévi-Strauss argues that the two levels of inquiry are complementary. As Edmund Leach puts it, Lévi-Strauss "holds that the study of history diachronically and the study of anthropology cross-culturally but synchronically are two alternative ways of doing the same kind of thing."[47]

Failure to draw a distinction similar to Mill's and Radcliffe-Brown's was a source of much confusion in the late nineteenth and early twentieth centuries: "The confusion that has reigned in the study of culture, which has delayed its progress, and which has of recent years caused much dissatisfaction to its students, is the result of a failure to consider sufficiently fully the methodology of the subject. The remedy is to recognize that the two different methods of explaining the facts of culture, the historical and the inductive, should be kept carefully separated in our minds."[48]

The work of John Dewey, a holist and a founder of psychological functionalism, certainly harbors this confusion, for he accepted a "principle of continuity" that subsumed without distinction both vertical and horizontal levels of inquiry. Dewey's acceptance of this principle dated back at least to the 1880's, when he was a neo-Hegelian still to be converted to pragmatism. In an 1888 work, Dewey praised the philosopher and mathematician G. W. Leibnitz for his organic view of the world and his emphasis on continuity: "Such thoughts as... that the universe is an interrelated unit; the thoughts of organism, of continuity, of uniformity of law—introduced and treated as Leibnitz treated them—are imperishable."[49]

It is worth looking at Leibnitz's interpretation of the principle of continuity in more detail. In a letter written in 1702, he explained: "To my mind everything is interconnected in the universe by virtue of metaphysical reasons so that *the present is always pregnant with the future*, and no given state is explicable naturally without reference to its immediately preceding state. If this be denied, the world will have hiatuses."[50] It is apparent that Leibnitz was interpreting the principle of continuity in what might be called a vertical or genetic sense: any given state was necessarily generated from the preceding state, and there were no gaps between them.

This vertical interpretation of continuity was reinforced in the two centuries after Leibnitz by the temporalization of the "Great Chain of Being," which had its origin in Greek thought. The idea had gradually developed that every type of thing that *could* exist *did* exist; thus there was a "chain" linking the most lowly at one end to the Creator at the other. However, during the eighteenth century the difficulties in this conception led to the chain's becoming temporalized; instead of being viewed as a static entity that had existed from the time of the creation, it was regarded as existing and developing within time.[51] This modification helped to prepare the way for Darwin; and publication of *The Origin of Species* in 1859 strengthened the belief that there was genetic continuity within nature. As Dewey once put it, "The philosophic significance of the doctrine of evolution lies precisely in its emphasis upon continuity of simpler and more complex organic forms until we reach man.... For the doctrine of organic development means that the living creature is a part of the world."[52]

Leibnitz, however, did not restrict himself to a vertical interpretation of the principle of continuity: "But as, according to my view, there is a perfect continuity reigning in the order of successive things *so there is a similar order in simultaneous things*, which fact establishes the plenum as real, and consigns empty spaces to imaginary realms. *In things existing simultaneously there may be continuity even though the imagination perceives only breaks.*"[53] This second interpretation could more accurately be termed a principle of horizontal interaction or interrelation than a principle of vertical continuity. Only confusion can result from both principles being loosely called "the principle of continuity."

The pertinent point is that Dewey's usage of the principle of continuity suffered from the same looseness. Like Leibnitz, he sometimes intended the term to signify the principle of genetic or vertical continuity between successive states, and at other times he meant the principle of horizontal interrelatedness or interconnection. It seems most likely that this looseness originated in Dewey's Hegelianism of the 1880's, for other neo-idealists of the late nineteenth and early twentieth centuries referred to the principle of continuity in the same two senses. A. E. Taylor, for example, began his short discussion of continuity in *Elements of Metaphysics* (1903) by referring to continuity within mathematical series. He quickly moved on to continuity of time series, followed by a jump from the vertical to the horizontal approach, with the continuity of causation as the center of interest. "Causation cannot possibly be thought of as discontinuous."[54] Later in the book, discussing the continuity of space, Taylor deliberately aimed "for the systematic establishment of the correspondence between the spatial and temporal series and the continuous series of real numbers."[55] F. H. Bradley also treated temporal and spatial continuity as though they had no significant differences.[56]

The principle of continuity as understood by the neo-idealists was related to the theory of internal (or "organic") relations, and can therefore be treated as part of the group of ideas forming Holism 1. Consider a situation where *A*, *B*, and *C* are externally, or mechanically, related entities—for example, three spatially related material entities (although some organicists would not regard this as an external relationship). It is possible in this case to separate *A* from *B* without altering the nature of *A*; and it is also possible to find a point where *A* ends and another where *B* or *C* begins. This is an example of discontinuity: *A*, *B*, and *C* are discrete and are only related externally.

By contrast, if there were continuity between *A*, *B*, and *C*, it would be impossible to find a point where *A* stopped or where *B* or *C* began.* This would occur in an organic whole where *A*, *B*, and *C* are internally related and the nature of each is determined in part by its relation to the others. To take a crude example, the heart and vascular system of a human can be regarded as organically interrelated and continuous; there is no place where the heart ends and the vascular system begins. Thus the principle of continuity as used in the late nineteenth and early twentieth centuries was related to the theory of internal relations, and hence to organicism, or Holism 1.

Dewey's confusion of vertical and horizontal continuity is illustrated by the variety of contexts in which he

---

* This followed from the "mathematical" definition of continuity, which was accepted by A. E. Taylor, and also by J. M. Baldwin and C. L. Fine in Baldwin's *Dictionary of Philosophy and Psychology* (1901).

postulates the existence of continuity without qualifying the term in any way. Continuity exists in the biological realm, for man is continuous with the animals, and the animals with chemical and physical processes. There are continuities between organism and environment, organism and organism (including man and man), mind and body, experience and nature, and subject and object. And experience itself forms a continuous stream.[57]

In Dewey's writings the themes of functionalism, evolutionism, organicism, and horizontal and vertical continuity come together. His essay "The Reflex Arc Concept in Psychology" (1896), which became the official starting point for American psychological functionalism, is a testament to Hegel as much as to Darwin and functional analysis. Here, Dewey argues that the reflex arc must be seen as a unified whole, a "coordination." Actually, he tends to depict a reflex circle rather than an arc. Here his organicism parallels that common among his contemporaries in biology and philosophy in the late nineteenth century. In referring to a circle, he is saying that in reflex action a stimulus interacts and coordinates with the response to it—in fact, is only a stimulus as such by virtue of the response—and that the response, similarly, only becomes a response by its coordination with the stimulus. Once again, William James's example of the husband being determined by the wife and the wife by the husband seems pertinent. Oblivious to this, Dewey writes in all seriousness: "What we have is a circuit, not an arc or broken segment of a circle. This circuit is more truly termed organic than reflex."[58]

The sociologist Don Martindale argues, "the true founders of functionalism were the positivistic organicists"; and his words are peculiarly applicable to Dewey, although he was not writing of psychological functionalism.[59] Martindale continues, in a passage that is fit to become, if not functionalism's epitaph, at least a warning for the unwary: "In ancient mythologies there sometimes appears the figure of a strange giant who gains his strength from contact with the earth. He is almost unbeatable by normal types of hand-to-hand combat, for when he is hurled to earth he gains strength from the contact and comes back with redoubled energy. In sociology, the organic point of view seems to have some of this property; cast down in the form of positivistic organicism, it arises with redoubled vigor in the form of functionalism."[60]

7

Holism and Psychology

IT IS PERHAPS a tribute to the importance of the science of psychology that it has already cropped up at several points in this discussion. But to do it justice, the focus of attention must again briefly return to the closing years of the nineteenth century.

During the 1890's there was a marked reaction within psychology to "the pure aggregative character of mental life which experimentalism had apparently demonstrated."[1] It is tempting to interpret this opposition to the "elementarist-associationist" (or analytic-reductionist) approach to psychology as a counterpart of the organicists' opposition to mechanistic analysis in biology, the idealist philosophers' reaction against mechanism and materialism, and the methodological holists' attacks on methodological individualism in history or sociology, all of which were contemporary with it.

By the early decades of the twentieth century the reactionary movement in psychology had given rise to functionalism, and also to Gestalt or configurationist psychology. The functionalists concentrated their attention on the problems of "how consciousness operates and what uses or functions it serves. The point of view they adopted was a Darwinian one in which the different operations of consciousness, sense perception, imagination, and emotion were all regarded as different instances of organic adaptation to the environment. Interest was thus directed to the overt behavior of the organism in relation to its environment as well as to the functioning of the mind."[2] Earlier it was mentioned that John Dewey's paper "The Reflex Arc Concept in Psychology" (1896) has usually been regarded as the foundation of functional psychology in the United States. Both Dewey and functionalism in general have already been discussed, so the second line of reaction in psychology against analysis and reductionism will be emphasized here.

Gestalt psychology had its origin in Max Wertheimer's paper "Perception of Apparent Movement" (1912), and it was developed further by the researches of Kurt Koffka and Wolfgang Köhler. Briefly, Gestalt psychologists applied the concept of wholeness to such areas of study as perception, behavior, and learning; they argued that in our mental life we are always dealing with *whole* objects or situations and not with mere aggregates of elements.

Köhler's *The Mentality of Apes* (1917) can be taken as an example of the Gestalt approach. Köhler worked on the principle that when his apes were placed in a situation requiring them to solve a problem, it was essential that the situation *as a whole* be apparent to them.

He criticized E. L. Thorndike's experiments for failing to provide the test animals with this total view: cats and dogs had been imprisoned in cages where they could not see the mechanisms that would release them, yet Thorndike was trying to make a psychological study of the processes that led to their escape.[3]

In 1920 Köhler developed his ideas further. He first defined the term "Gestalts" and his definition clearly showed the similarity between Gestalt psychology and organicism: "When spatial, visual, auditory, and intellectual processes are such as to display properties other than could be derived from the parts in summation, they may be regarded as unities illustrating what we mean by the word 'Gestalts.' "[4] Köhler then pointed out that the use of the Gestalt concept apparently marked psychology off from the natural sciences; indeed, the suspicion was that a search for Gestalts in other fields "would somehow violate the fundamentals of exact science."[5]

Köhler nevertheless proceeded, apparently successfully, to search for Gestalts in the physical sciences. One example he cites is the distribution of electrostatic charge over the surface of a conductor.[6] The distribution of the charge cannot be viewed satisfactorily as an aggregate of charges on small areas of the conductor; the whole has to be taken into account. But Köhler overlooks an important fact. His example is an electrostatic field, and it is true that in such a field the situation as a whole has to be taken into account; but this is no indication that the analytic or summative method has failed. On the contrary, it was by using the analytic method over a long period that physical scientists established formulae to accurately describe the interaction between elements of electrical, magnetic, or gravitational fields, and the formulae themselves indicate why the whole field must be considered.

Some writers have argued that the situation with respect to so-called field theories in psychology is quite different. The attempt to find parallels between physics and psychology in terms of fields (in the manner of the Gestalt theorists or Kurt Lewin) is called a "fad" by Gustav Bergmann, who adds: "It is absurd at the present stage of psychological knowledge. I don't think that the extra caution is necessary. However that may be, the proponents of psychological field theory behaved as if trying to benefit from the prestige of field theories in physics by usurping an attractive label for their particular ideas. This motive may have been unconscious."[7]

One serious complication emerges here to prevent, or at least delay, the identification of the Gestalt psychologists as supporters of Holism 1. At one point Köhler specifically discusses what has been called philosophical organicism, and his only criticism appears to be that it is rather general and indefinite: "One point of view would be that nature is composed of independent elements whose purely additive total constitutes reality. Another that there are no such elements in nature, that all states and processes are real in a vast universal whole, and hence that all 'parts' are but products of abstraction. The first proposition is completely wrong; the second hinders comprehension of the Gestalt principle more than it helps. . . . If natural science has never been greatly concerned with the doctrine of universal interactionism, philosophy, unhampered by concrete examples of physical phenomena, has suffered all the more. The doctrine appears to be a complete acceptance of the Gestalt principle; in point of fact it only corrupts that principle. The trouble is, no one can take so general and indefinite an hypothesis seriously."[8] From this passage it would seem that Köhler was an organicist, but that he sought in some way for a less "corrupt" form of the theory. Certainly he was an opponent of the "additive" (i.e. analytic) method.

However, Köhler's words a little later give a different perspective: "The concepts of parts, of summations, etc., do not lose their important significance when we deal with Gestalt phenomena. One must be clear, however, about what it is to which the concepts are applied."[9] The point suggested here can be developed and expressed— though in a way that Köhler might not have endorsed— in terms of visual perception. Consider a crude form of Max Wertheimer's 1912 experiment: we see two flashing lights, A and B, which are spatially separated but which, if seen to flash at less than a certain time interval, give rise to the sensation that a light is actually moving from point A to point B. In considering the virtues of the analytic method as opposed to organicism in this case, great care must be taken, as Köhler points out, to define *what* it is to which our concepts are applied.

In the first place, there is the physical situation, a system of two flashing lights that are spatially separated. In this case, the system, or whole, can be investigated using the analytic method. But there is a second system, namely, the experience of the observer. He does not see *two* spatially separated flashing lights, so from the point of view of his experience these are not the elements. All he experiences is a light that moves from point A to point B; and it is *this* whole that must be analyzed into its elements (light starting at A, movement, light ending at B). It would be a serious confusion to take the elements of the physical situation and suppose that by some sort of addition they result in perceived movement; this would be to take the elements of one whole as the elements of a different whole.

Another way of approaching this is to argue that it is up to empirical research (coupled, of course, with theoretical endeavor) to reveal the laws pertaining to human perception—that is, how physical systems will be perceived under various conditions. There is nothing logically reprehensible in arguing that under certain conditions even a simple set of physical elements can give rise to the most surprising visual phenomena. Possibly this was what Köhler was trying to express when he wrote: "The Gestalt laws observed by such phenomena and the specific structure spontaneously and objectively assumed *prescribe for us* what we are to recognize 'as one thing.'"[10]

If Gestalt principles are concerned with how one system (e.g. the physical realm) relates to another (e.g. what it is that is perceived), then they cannot be criticized as being holistic in the objectionable sense. And there is much in Gestalt psychology that is concerned with just this—for example, Wertheimer's principles of perceptual organization (one of which is the principle of proximity: parts that are close together in time or space tend to be perceived together).

The Gestalt psychologists cannot be completely exonerated, however. As shown earlier, there are passages in Köhler that have a familiar organicist ring; and Edward H. Madden has found the same in the writings of Koffka and Wertheimer.[11] Making a distinction between *W* Gestalts (systems that determine the nature of their parts) and *K* Gestalts (systems marked by functional interrelationships between their parts), Madden has clarified just what Wertheimer was asserting when he held that "the whole is more than the sum of the parts." Madden argues that all the valid parts of the Gestalt position can be expressed in analytical terminology.

In Madden's view, the crux of the matter is that in rejecting the analytic method Köhler, Koffka, and Wertheimer overlook the fact that when the initial conditions of a system are described, not only the qualities or conditions of the parts are included, but also the network of relational qualities. This is true even in classical Newtonian examples, as Madden shows. For example, in a mechanistic system composed of a number of specified objects, the objects' positions and velocities (both relational features pertinent to the way in which the objects interact) are as much a part of the initial conditions as the masses of the objects. In fact, the laws that are known to apply will determine the relevant initial conditions. Madden concludes: "What the Gestalters wish to say in their characteristic way about science can be said more clearly in the ordinary, analytical way which they reject as in principle inadequate. Some of what they actually do say in their own characteristic way turns out to be misleading."[12]

Other areas of psychology in which holistic ideas sometimes appear have not yet been mentioned. These include social psychology, genetic psychology, psychiatry, and an amalgam of all these, the so-called humanistic psychology. A recent book of readings in this last field groups its first four contributions in a section titled "The whole is greater than the part."[13] The first of these four papers, by J. F. T. Bugental, begins with an attack on "the model of man as a composite of part functions" and "the model of a science taken over from physics."[14] The following paper, by Abraham Maslow, reports: "The lessons of Gestalt psychology and of organismic theory have not been fully integrated into psychology. The human being is an irreducible unit, at least as far as psychological research is concerned. Everything in him is related to everything else, in greater or lesser degree."[15]

As another example, consider Kurt Goldstein's book *The Organism* (1939), which Robert Woodworth discusses as "organismic psychology" in the later editions of his *Contemporary Schools of Psychology*,[16] and which Maslow and others recognize as a precursor of contemporary humanistic psychology. Goldstein uses material from medicine, biology, neurology, psychology, and psychiatry to support what he terms "the so-called ho-

listic, organismic approach."[17] Much of this holistic
framework is intended to emphasize the interrelationship between the processes taking place in various parts
of the human organism—in other words, to make a point
that supporters of the analytic method would not necessarily disagree with, namely, that man is in a sense a
"functional whole."

However, Goldstein's holism did become objectionable when it led him—in the manner of the humanistic
psychologists—to charge what he variously called the
"dissecting method of natural science" or the "atomistic
approach" with being in principle an unsuitable method
of investigation:[18] "Yet ultimately our procedure is root-
ed in a more profound conviction: *this is the conviction
that a state of greater perfection can never be understood
from that of less perfection, and that only the converse
is possible.* It is very feasible to isolate parts from a whole,
but a perfect whole can never be composed by synthesiz-
ing it from the less perfect parts."[19]

The wheel has turned full circle, for it was with the
investigation of this charge that the present book opened.

Postscript

OUR DISCUSSION of holism opened with a quotation from Arthur O. Lovejoy, and it is appropriate to refer back to this by way of conclusion. For the thesis that has been argued in the foregoing pages is that significant numbers of the contemporary generation of human scientists have had their thinking determined by the holistic "turn of reasoning, trick of logic, methodological assumption," which is indeed "highly debatable."

Not that the problems with which modern holists have been concerned are unimportant. The best method of investigating organic wholes, the effects of analytic decomposition, the types of concepts that are fruitful in discussing the properties of wholes, and so on, are all highly significant and complex questions. Nor has it been claimed that the holists have been entirely mistaken. They have been right to emphasize the dynamic relation between the parts of an organic whole (Holism 1); they have been right to point to the difficulty in predicting beforehand the emergent properties that result when new elements are brought into combination; and they have been right to stress that the scientific discussion of organic wholes would be facilitated by the introduction of new concepts into the vocabulary of the sciences (Holism 3).

Where the holists have been wrong is in thinking that there is anything here that is antithetical to the traditional analytic (or atomistic, or mechanistic) method. Their errors in this area can be traced to a failure to give an adequate account of this method and to their willingness to accept an oversimplified view of traditional science. Moreover, they have been blind to the difference between emergence and reductionism, a shortcoming probably attributable to a lingering affection for Hegel's principle of internal relations and the organicism to which it gives rise.

In short, the analytic or mechanistic method, in the form expounded by such writers as Madden, Hempel, and Nagel, is such a moderate and reasonable position that no scientist, not even a holist, can avoid putting it into practice. By contrast, holism—taken seriously—is an eminently unworkable doctrine.

Notes

Notes

Complete authors' names, titles, and publishing information for sources cited in the Notes will be found in the Bibliography, pp. 135–44.

Chapter 1

1. Bradley, p. 18; but cf. p. 514.
2. *Ibid.*, pp. 513–19.
3. *Ibid.*, pp. 518–19.
4. Hegel, *Science of Logic*, II, 350. See also Moore, "External and Internal Relations," esp. p. 284.
5. McTaggart, I, 113.
6. This seems to be the substance of G. E. Moore's attacks on internal relations. See Moore, "External and Internal Relations," p. 284, and *Principia Ethica*, p. 33.
7. Defining and accompanying characteristics are discussed in John Hospers, Chapter 1.
8. L. Wittgenstein, *Philosophical Investigations* (tr. G. E. M. Anscombe; Oxford University Press, 1963), Sections 66–67.
9. Russell, p. 772.
10. Nagel, *Structure of Science*, pp. 438, 442–43.
11. Nagel, "Mechanistic Explanation and Organismic Biology," p. 136.
12. Nagel, *Structure of Science*, pp. 372–73.
13. Moore, *Principia Ethica*, p. 33.
14. McTaggart, p. 161. My emphasis.
15. Taylor, pp. 113–14.
16. McTaggart, pp. 112–13.
17. *Ibid.*, p. 119.

Chapter 2

1. Blending inheritance is discussed by E. B. Gasking, *Scientific Investigation of Generation, 1650–1910* (Ph.D. thesis, University of Melbourne, 1962); and also by Gavin de Beer, *Charles Darwin* (London, 1963).

2. Haldane, *The Sciences and Philosophy*, p. 219.

3. See, for example, Driesch, *The Science and Philosophy of the Organism*.

4. Rudolf Virchow, *Disease, Life and Man: Selected Essays of Rudolf Virchow* (tr. Lelland J. Rather; Stanford, Calif., 1959), p. 106.

5. As an example, see Schubert-Soldern, *Mechanism and Vitalism*.

6. Haldane, *The Sciences and Philosophy*, pp. 74–75.

7. Bertalanffy, *Modern Theories of Development*, p. 9.

8. R. B. and J. S. Haldane, "The Relation of Philosophy to Science," in Seth and Haldane, p. 56.

9. Haldane, "Life and Mechanism," p. 35.

10. *Ibid.*, p. 31.

11. *Ibid.*, p. 38.

12. See Keeton, "Edmund Montgomery: A Pioneer of Organicism."

13. Montgomery, "Unity of the Organic Individual," p. 326. See also his "Are We Cell-Aggregates?"

14. Haldane, "Life and Mechanism," p. 33.

Chapter 3

1. The conference proceedings appear in Koestler and Smythies, *Beyond Reductionism: The Alpbach Symposium*.

2. Weiss, "$1 + 1 \neq 2$," p. 802.

3. *Ibid.*

4. *Ibid.*, p. 814. Weiss's antireductionism is also discussed in Pratt, pp. 1–16.

5. Weiss, "The Living System," p. 9. My emphasis.

6. *Ibid.*, pp. 9–10.

7. Weiss, "$1 + 1 \neq 2$," p. 819.

8. Weiss, "The Living System," p. 42.

9. Durkheim, pp. 97–98. It should be noted that many individualists—including Popper, Watkins, and Agassi—object to
the stress on psychology that is found here.

10. Watkins, "Historical Explanation," p. 504.

11. *Ibid.*, p. 505.

12. Durkheim, p. 101.

13. *Ibid.*, p. 102.

14. Watkins, "Historical Explanation," p. 505.

15. Mandelbaum, "Societal Facts," pp. 478–79.

16. *Ibid.*, p. 480.

17. Watkins, "Historical Explanation," p. 506n.

18. Agassi, pp. 244–45.

19. Hayek, p. 41.

20. *Ibid.*, p. 42.

21. Watkins, "Historical Explanation," p. 505.

22. Watkins, "Ideal Types," p. 731.

23. Popper, *The Open Society*, p. 98.

24. Bertalanffy, *Modern Theories of Development*, p. 46.

25. Bertalanffy, *Problems of Life*, p. 199.

26. Bertalanffy, "Chance or Law," p. 56.

Chapter 4

1. Bertalanffy, *General System Theory*, p. 22. See also his
Modern Theories of Development, p. 46.

2. Bertalanffy, *General System Theory*, pp. 18–19.

3. *Ibid.*, p. 37. See also Bertalanffy, *Problems of Life*, p. 199.

4. Angyal, "A Logic of Systems," reprinted in Emery, p. 26.

5. See Phillips, "John Dewey and the Organismic Archetype."

6. Dewey, "The New Psychology," *Andover Review*, II
(1884), 285.

7. Dewey and Bentley, "Interaction and Transaction," p. 506.

8. *Ibid.*, p. 509. The authors used hyphens to accentuate the
significance of the terms used.

9. *Ibid.*

10. Dewey and Bentley, "Transactions as Known and Named,"
p. 533.

11. *Ibid.*, p. 536.

12. *Ibid.*, p. 547.

13. James, "Absolutism and Empiricism," pp. 282–83. My emphasis.
14. Dewey and Bentley, "Transactions," p. 547.
15. Bertalanffy, *Problems of Life,* pp. 11–12.
16. See Hospers, Chapter 1.
17. Nagel, "Mechanistic Explanation," p. 138.
18. Dewey and Bentley, "Transactions," p. 547.
19. Nagel, "Mechanistic Explanation," pp. 140–41.
20. Bertalanffy, *General System Theory,* p. 19.
21. *Ibid.,* p. 23.
22. Anatol Rapoport, Foreword to Buckley, *Modern Systems Research,* p. xvii.
23. R. L. Ackoff, "Systems, Organizations, and Interdisciplinary Research," in Eckman, pp. 27–28.
24. As quoted by Ralph Barton Perry, *The Thought and Character of William James* (Oxford University Press, 1935), I, 482. James was in fact repeating an attack that had been made on the ideas of Herbert Spencer.
25. This is proposed by Hall and Fagen; see particularly their p. 82.
26. Bertalanffy, *Problems of Life,* p. 199.
27. For example, Kenneth E. Boulding, "General Systems Theory: The Skeleton of Science," in Buckley, *Modern Systems Research.*
28. See Buckley, *Modern Systems Research,* Parts II and III.
29. Bertalanffy, "General System Theory: A Critical Review," *ibid.,* p. 13.
30. Popper, *The Logic of Scientific Discovery.*
31. Bertalanffy, in Buckley, *Modern Systems Research,* p. 21.

Chapter 5

1. Koestler, p. 61.
2. *Ibid.,* p. 45.
3. *Ibid.,* p. 48.
4. *Ibid.*
5. *Ibid.,* Chapter 2.
6. *Ibid.,* p. 41.
7. *Ibid.,* p. 348.
8. *Ibid.,* pp. 45–47.
9. *Ibid.,* p. 54.
10. See Easton, *A Framework for Political Analysis* and *A Systems Analysis of Political Life.*

11. *American Political Science Review*, LXI (1967), 157.
12. Easton, *A Framework for Political Analysis*, p. 23.
13. Beer, in Eckman, pp. 18–19.
14. Easton, *A Framework for Political Analysis*, p. 27.
15. These arguments appear *ibid.*, pp. 29–30.
16. *Ibid.*, p. 31.
17. Easton, *A Systems Analysis of Political Life*, p. 479.

Chapter 6

1. Jonathan Culler, "The Linguistic Basis of Structuralism," in Robey, p. 20.
2. Lévi-Strauss, p. 21.
3. See Lane, p. 14.
4. John Mepham, "The Structuralist Sciences and Philosophy," in Robey, p. 108.
5. Lévi-Strauss, p. 33. His emphasis.
6. Piaget, *Structuralism*, p. 5.
7. Lévi-Strauss, p. 37. For a critique of Lévi-Strauss's views on kinship, see Leach, Chapter 6.
8. See Lévi-Strauss, p. 39. 9. *Ibid.*, p. 41.
10. *Ibid.* 11. *Ibid.*, p. 42.
12. Boudon, p. 13. 13. Lévi-Strauss, p. 46.
14. *Ibid.*, p. 212.
15. Piaget, *Structuralism*, p. 4.
16. Kallen, p. 523.
17. See J. A. Lauwerys, "Herbert Spencer and the Scientific Movement," in A. V. Judges, ed., *Pioneers of English Education* (London, 1952).
18. See Phillips, "The Idea of Evolution in Educational Thought."
19. Spencer, *Essays on Education*, p. 175.
20. Spencer, *First Principles*, p. 358.
21. Spencer, *Principles of Sociology*, p. 459.
22. *Ibid.*, p. 473. 23. *Ibid.*, pp. 459–61.
24. *Ibid.*, p. 461. 25. *Ibid.*, p. 463.
26. Hempel, p. 185. 27. *Ibid.*, p. 210.
28. *Ibid.*, p. 206.
29. Ryan, *Philosophy of the Social Sciences*, p. 173.

30. Catton, p. 91.
31. Hempel, p. 191.
32. James, *Talks to Teachers*, pp. 13–15.
33. Merton, p. 51.   34. *Ibid.*, p. 31.
35. Kallen, p. 523.   36. Catton, p. 75.
37. Ryan, *Philosophy of the Social Sciences*, p. 193.
38. Merton, p. 47.
39. *Ibid.*, p. 27.
40. Sigmund Freud, "The Question of Lay-Analysis," in *Two Short Accounts of Psycho-Analysis* (Harmondsworth, 1970), p. 113.
41. Mill, pp. 343–44.
42. Popper, *The Poverty of Historicism*, p. 143.
43. *Ibid.*, p. 117.
44. Piaget, *Structuralism*, p. 107.
45. Radcliffe-Brown, p. 40.
46. *Ibid.*, pp. 40–41.
47. Leach, p. 15.
48. Radcliffe-Brown, pp. 24–25.
49. Dewey, *Leibniz's New Essays*, p. 272.
50. Leibnitz, p. 185. Emphasis in original.
51. See Lovejoy, *The Great Chain of Being*.
52. Dewey, *Democracy and Education*, pp. 392–93.
53. Leibnitz, p. 186. My emphasis.
54. Taylor, p. 173.
55. *Ibid.*, p. 248.
56. See Bradley, Chapters 4–6.
57. Phillips, "John Dewey and the Organismic Archetype," pp. 251–54.
58. Dewey, "The Reflex Arc," p. 363.
59. Martindale, p. 448.
60. *Ibid.*, p. 449.

Chapter 7

1. Hartmann, p. 16. Many historians of psychology have made similar comments.
2. Spence, p. 147.
3. Köhler, *Mentality of Apes*, esp. p. 27.

4. Köhler, "Physical Gestalten," p. 513.
5. *Ibid.*
6. *Ibid.*, pp. 521–24.
7. Bergmann, p. 11.
8. Köhler, "Physical Gestalten," p. 525.
9. *Ibid.*, p. 526.
10. *Ibid.*, p. 527. Köhler's emphasis.
11. Madden, *Philosophical Problems of Psychology*, esp. Chapter 1.
12. *Ibid.*, p. 24.
13. See Severin, *Humanistic Viewpoints in Psychology: A Book of Readings.*
14. *Ibid.*, pp. 8–9.
15. *Ibid.*, p. 32.
16. See Woodworth, Chapter 7.
17. Goldstein, p. vi.
18. *Ibid.*, pp. vi, 514.
19. *Ibid.*, p. 515. His emphasis.

Bibliography

The literature pertaining to holism is enormous, as the sampling in this listing might imply. It therefore seems worthwhile to indicate a few sources that are particularly useful or are convenient starting points for further investigation, although it is hoped that the sources cited throughout the book will already have aided the reader in this respect.

A detailed discussion of the analytic or mechanistic method of scientific investigation, of organicism, and of reductionism can be found in Ernest Nagel, *The Structure of Science*. The symposium edited by Marjorie Grene, *Interpretations of Life and Mind*, raises other issues about reductionism, as does the paper by Vernon Pratt, "Explaining the Properties of Organisms." Also worth consulting on this topic are Arthur Koestler and J. R. Smythies, *Beyond Reductionism*, and F. J. Ayala and T. Dobzhansky, *Studies in the Philosophy of Biology*. Other aspects of the philosophy of social science are addressed in May Brodbeck, ed., *Readings in the Philosophy of the Social Sciences* (New York, 1969); of special interest in this volume is Carl G. Hempel's paper on functionalism.

Hegel's work has been subject to intensive discussion recently, and several introductory works and "reinterpretations" have appeared. A two-part review of current scholarship is given by Anthony Quinton in *The New York Review of Books*, XXII (1975), Nos. 9 and 10. Quinton's own *Absolute Idealism* is clear. Far more readable than Hegel for those wishing to capture something of the flavor of nineteenth-century idealism is F. H. Bradley's *Appearance and Reality*.

Many of the papers in the dispute between the methodological individualists and the holists have been collected in an anthology by John O'Neill, *Modes of Individualism and Collectivism*, which also presents a good bibliography. The book edited by Alan Ryan, *The Philosophy of Social Explanation*, includes several of these papers, together with others on structuralism and functionalism.

Of the many books on General System Theory, probably the most useful—owing to the broad range of authors represented— is Walter Buckley, ed., *Modern Systems Research for the Behavioral Scientist*. More recently, a symposium on the subject appeared in *The Academy of Management Journal*, XV, December 1972. The classic work is probably Ludwig von Bertalanffy's *General System Theory*.

Two valuable collections on structuralism are David Robey's *Structuralism: An Introduction*, and Michael Lane's *Introduction to Structuralism*. A readable guide to the work of Lévi-Strauss is Edmund Leach, *Lévi-Strauss*.

Edward H. Madden's critical analysis of the holistic claims of Gestalt psychologists will be found in his *Philosophical Problems of Psychology*; and some of the claims themselves appear in Wolfgang Köhler, *Gestalt Psychology*. Many of the major writers in the humanistic psychology movement, and some others, are represented in Frank T. Severin, ed., *Humanistic Viewpoints in Psychology*.

Ackoff, Russell L., and Fred E. Emery. *On Purposeful Systems.* London, 1972.

Agassi, Joseph. "Methodological Individualism," *British Journal of Sociology*, 11 (1960).

Alexander, Samuel. *Space, Time, and Deity.* London, 1920.

Angyal, Andras. *Foundations for a Science of Personality.* New York, 1941.

Ansbacher, H. L. "On the Origin of Holism," *Journal of Individual Psychology*, XVII (1961).

Arnheim, R. *Visual Thinking.* Berkeley, Calif., 1969.

Bibliography

Ayala, F. J., and T. Dobzhansky, eds. *Studies in the Philosophy of Biology*. Berkeley, Calif., 1974.

Barnes, Harry Elmer. "Representative Biological Theories of Society," *Sociological Review*, XVII (1925).

Beckner, M. *The Biological Way of Thought*. Berkeley, Calif., 1968.

Bergmann, Gustav. *Philosophy of Science*. Madison, Wisc., 1957.

Bertalanffy, Ludwig von. "Chance or Law," *in* Koestler and Smythies, *Beyond Reductionism*.

—— *General System Theory: Foundations, Development, Applications*. New York, 1969.

—— "The History and Status of General Systems Theory," *Academy of Management Journal*, XV (1972).

—— *Modern Theories of Development* (tr. J. H. Woodger). New York, 1962.

—— *Problems of Life*. New York, 1960.

Boudon, Raymond. *The Uses of Structuralism* (tr. Michalina Vaughan). London, 1971.

Bradley, F. H. *Appearance and Reality* (2d ed.). Oxford University Press, 1962.

Brodbeck, May. "Methodological Individualisms: Definition and Reduction," *Philosophy of Science*, XXV (1958).

Buckley, Walter, ed. *Modern Systems Research for the Behavioral Scientist*. Chicago, 1968.

—— *Sociology and Modern Systems Theory*. Englewood Cliffs, N.J., 1967.

Cannon, Walter B. *The Wisdom of the Body* (rev. ed.). New York, 1939.

Catton, William R., Jr. *From Animistic to Naturalistic Sociology*. New York, 1966.

Churchman, C. West. *The Systems Approach*. New York, 1968.

Coker, F. W. *Organismic Theories of the State*. New York, 1910.

Commins, W. D. "Some Early Holistic Psychologists," *Journal of Philosophy*, XXIX (1932).

Coombs, Philip H. *The World Educational Crisis: A Systems Analysis*. New York, 1968.

Dagenais, James J. *Models of Man: A Phenomenological Critique of Some Paradigms in the Human Sciences*. The Hague, 1972.

Bibliography

Demerath, N. J., and R. Peterson, eds. *System, Change and Conflict: A Reader on Contemporary Sociological Theory and the Debate over Functionalism.* New York, 1967.

Dewey, John. "Body and Mind," *in* John Dewey, *Philosophy and Civilization.* New York, 1931.

—— *Democracy and Education.* New York, 1958.

—— *Leibniz's New Essays Concerning the Human Understanding.* Chicago, 1888.

—— "The New Psychology," *Andover Review,* II (1884).

—— "The Reflex Arc Concept in Psychology," *Psychological Review,* III (1896).

—— "Social as a Category," *The Monist,* XXXVIII (1928).

—— "The Unity of the Human Being," *in* Joseph Ratner, ed., *Intelligence in the Modern World.* New York, 1939.

Dewey, John, and Arthur F. Bentley. "Interaction and Transaction," *Journal of Philosophy,* XLIII (1946).

—— "Transactions as Known and Named," *Journal of Philosophy,* XLIII (1946).

Diesing, Paul. *Patterns of Discovery in the Social Sciences.* London, 1972.

Dogan, Mattei, and Stein Rokkan, eds. *Quantitative Ecological Analysis in the Social Sciences.* Cambridge, Mass., 1969.

Driesch, Hans. *The Science and Philosophy of the Organism.* London, 1908.

Durkheim, Emile. *The Rules of Sociological Method* (8th ed., tr. Sarah Solovay and John Mueller). New York, 1964.

Easton, David. *A Framework for Political Analysis.* Englewood Cliffs, N.J., 1965.

—— *A Systems Analysis of Political Life.* New York, 1965.

Eckman, Donald P., ed. *Systems: Research and Design.* New York, 1961.

Ehrmann, Jacques, ed. *Structuralism.* New York, 1970.

Emery, F. E., ed. *Systems Thinking.* Harmondsworth, 1970.

Emmet, Dorothy. *Whitehead's Philosophy of Organism* (2d ed.). London, 1966.

Findlay, J. N. *Hegel: A Re-examination.* London, 1958.

Fuller, R. Buckminster. *Operating Manual for Spaceship Earth.* New York, 1970.

Bibliography

Gellner, Ernest. "Holism versus Individualism in History and Sociology," *in* Patrick Gardiner, ed., *Theories of History*. New York, 1959.

Ginsberg, Morris. "The Individual and Society," *in* M. Ginsberg, *On the Diversity of Morals*. London, 1956.

Goldstein, Kurt. *The Organism*. Boston, 1963.

Goldstein, Leon J. "The Inadequacy of the Principle of Methodological Individualism," *Journal of Philosophy*, LIII (1956).

—— "Two Theses of Methodological Individualism," *British Journal for the Philosophy of Science*, IX (1958).

Gray, W., F. D. Duhl, and N. D. Rizzo, eds. *General Systems Theory and Psychiatry*. Boston, 1968.

Gray, W., and N. D. Rizzo, eds. *Unity Through Diversity: Festschrift in Honor of Ludwig von Bertalanffy*. New York, 1971.

Grene, Marjorie, ed. *Interpretations of Life and Mind*. New York, 1971.

Haldane, J. S. "Life and Mechanism," *Mind*, IX (1884).

—— *The Sciences and Philosophy*. London, 1929.

Hall, A. D., and R. E. Fagen. "Definition of System," *in* Buckley, *Modern Systems Research*.

Hartmann, George W. *Gestalt Psychology*. New York, 1935.

Hayek, F. A. von. "Scientism and the Study of Society, Part 2," *Economica*, X (1943).

Hegel, G. W. F. *The Philosophy of History* (tr. J. Sibree). New York, 1956.

—— *The Science of Logic* (tr. W. H. Johnson and L. G. Struthers). New York, 1929.

Hempel, Carl G. "The Logic of Functional Analysis," *in* May Brodbeck, ed., *Readings in the Philosophy of the Social Sciences*. New York, 1969.

Hospers, John. *An Introduction to Philosophical Analysis* (rev. ed.). London, 1967.

James, William. "Absolutism and Empiricism," *Mind*, IX (1884).

—— *Talks to Teachers on Psychology*. London, 1925.

Kallen, Horace. "Functionalism," *in* E. Seligman and A. Johnson, eds., *Encyclopedia of the Social Sciences*, Vol. 6. New York, 1959.

[139]

Bibliography

Kast, Fremont E., and James E. Rosenzweig. "General Systems Theory: Applications for Organization and Management," *Academy of Management Journal,* XV (1972).

Keeton, Morris T. "Edmund Montgomery: A Pioneer of Organicism," *Journal of the History of Ideas,* VIII (1947).

Koestler, Arthur. *The Ghost in the Machine.* London, 1967.

Koestler, Arthur, and J. R. Smythies, eds. *Beyond Reductionism: The Alpbach Symposium.* London, 1972.

Köhler, Wolfgang. *Gestalt Psychology.* New York, 1947.

—— *The Mentality of Apes* (tr. Ella Winter). Harmondsworth, 1957.

—— "Physical Gestalten," *in* Wayne Dennis, ed., *Readings in the History of Psychology.* New York, 1948.

Laing, R. D. *The Divided Self.* Harmondsworth, 1965.

Lane, Michael, ed. *Introduction to Structuralism.* New York, 1973.

Laszlo, Ervin. *Introduction to Systems Philosophy.* New York, 1971.

—— *The Relevance of General Systems Theory.* New York, 1972.

—— *The Systems View of the World.* New York, 1972.

Leach, Edmund. *Lévi-Strauss.* London, 1970.

Lee, Alfred McClung. "The Concept of System," *Social Research,* XXXII (1965).

Leibnitz, G. W. F. *Leibniz Selections* (ed. P. P. Wiener). New York, 1951.

Lerner, Daniel, ed. *Parts and Wholes.* New York, 1963.

Lévi-Strauss, Claude. *Structural Anthropology* (tr. Claire Jacobson and Brooke Grundfest Schoepf). Harmondsworth, 1972.

Lossky, N. O. *The World as an Organic Whole* (tr. Natalie Duddington). Oxford University Press, 1928.

Lovejoy, Arthur O. *The Great Chain of Being.* New York, 1960.

Lukes, Stephen. "Methodological Individualism Reconsidered," *in* Dorothy Emmet and Alasdair MacIntyre, eds., *Sociological Theory and Philosophical Analysis.* London, 1970.

McTaggart, J. *The Nature of Existence.* Cambridge, Eng., 1921.

Madden, Edward H. *Philosophical Problems of Psychology.* New York, 1962.

Bibliography

———— "The Philosophy of Science in Gestalt Theory," *in* H. Feigl and M. Brodbeck, eds., *Readings in the Philosophy of Science*. New York, 1953.

Mandelbaum, Maurice. *History, Man, and Reason: A Study in Nineteenth-Century Thought*. Baltimore, 1971.

———— "Societal Facts," *in* Patrick Gardiner, ed., *Theories of History*. New York, 1959.

———— "Societal Laws," *British Journal for the Philosophy of Science*, VIII (1957).

Manuel, Frank E. "From Equality to Organicism," *Journal of the History of Ideas*, XVII (1956).

Martindale, Don. *The Nature and Types of Sociological Theory*. London, 1967.

Maslow, Abraham H. *Religions, Values, and Peak Experiences*. New York, 1970.

May, Rollo, ed. *Existential Psychology* (2d ed.). New York, 1969.

Merton, Robert K. *Social Theory and Social Structure*. New York, 1957.

Milholland, F., and B. E. Forisha. *From Skinner to Rogers*. Lincoln, Neb., 1973.

Mill, John Stuart. *Philosophy of Scientific Method* (ed. Ernest Nagel). New York, 1950.

Miller, James G. *Living Systems*. New York, 1972.

———— "Living Systems: Basic Concepts," *Behavioral Science*, X (1965).

———— "Living Systems: The Organization," *Behavioral Science*, XVII (1972).

———— "Toward a General Theory for the Behavioral Sciences," *American Psychologist*, X (1955).

Montgomery, Edmund. "Are We Cell-Aggregates?," *Mind*, VII (1882).

———— "The Unity of the Organic Individual," *Mind*, V (1880).

Moore, G. E. "External and Internal Relations," *in* Moore, *Philosophical Studies*. London, 1960.

———— *Principia Ethica*. Cambridge, Eng., 1970.

Morgan, C. Lloyd. "A Concept of the Organism, Emergent and Resultant," *Proceedings of the Aristotelian Society* (N.S.), XXVII (1926–27).

Bibliography

Nagel, Ernest. "Mechanistic Explanation and Organismic Biology," *in* E. H. Madden, ed., *The Structure of Scientific Thought*. Boston, 1960.

—— *The Structure of Science*. London, 1961.

O'Neill, John, ed. *Modes of Individualism and Collectivism*. London, 1973.

Parascandola, John. "Organismic and Holistic Concepts in the Thought of L. J. Henderson," *Journal of the History of Biology*, IV (1971).

Peery, Newman S., Jr. "General Systems Theory: An Inquiry into Its Social Philosophy," *Academy of Management Journal*, XV (1972).

Pepper, Stephen C. *World Hypotheses*. Berkeley, Calif., 1957.

Phillips, D. C. "The Idea of Evolution in Educational Thought," *in* E. L. French, ed., *Melbourne Studies in Education, 1965*. Melbourne, 1966.

—— "James, Dewey, and the Reflex Arc," *Journal of the History of Ideas*, XXXII (1971).

—— "John Dewey and the Organismic Archetype," *in* R. J. W. Selleck, ed., *Melbourne Studies in Education, 1971*. Melbourne, 1971.

—— "The Methodological Basis of Systems Theory," *Academy of Management Journal*, XV (1972).

—— "Organicism in the Late Nineteenth and Early Twentieth Centuries," *Journal of the History of Ideas*, XXXI (1970).

—— "Systems Theory: A Discredited Philosophy," *Abacus*, V (1969).

Piaget, Jean. *Main Trends in Interdisciplinary Research*. New York, 1973.

—— *Structuralism* (tr. Chaninah Maschler). London, 1971.

Popper, Karl R. *The Logic of Scientific Discovery*. London, 1965.

—— *The Open Society and Its Enemies*. London, 1969.

—— *The Poverty of Historicism*. London, 1969.

Pratt, Vernon. "Explaining the Properties of Organisms," *Studies in History and Philosophy of Science*, V (1974).

Quinton, Anthony M. *Absolute Idealism*. Oxford University Press, 1972.

Bibliography

Radcliffe-Brown, A. R. *Method in Social Anthropology* (ed. M. N. Srinivas). Chicago, 1958.

Robey, David, ed. *Structuralism: An Introduction. Wolfson College Lectures, 1972.* Oxford University Press, 1973.

Rogers, Carl. *Freedom to Learn.* Columbus, O., 1969.

Royce, Josiah. *The Spirit of Modern Philosophy.* Boston, 1892.

Russell, Bertrand. *A History of Western Philosophy.* London, 1948.

Ryan, Alan, ed. *The Philosophy of Social Explanation.* Oxford University Press, 1973.

——— *The Philosophy of the Social Sciences.* London, 1970.

Salmon, G. "Social Organism," *in* E. Seligman and A. Johnson, eds., *Encyclopedia of the Social Sciences*, Vol. 14. New York, 1934.

Schubert-Soldern, Rainier. *Mechanism and Vitalism* (ed. P. G. Fothergill, tr. C. E. Robin). London, 1962.

Scott, K. J. "Methodological and Epistemological Individualism," *British Journal for the Philosophy of Science*, XI (1961).

Sellars, Roy Wood. *Evolutionary Naturalism.* Chicago, 1922.

Seth, Andrew, and R. B. Haldane, eds. *Essays in Philosophical Criticism.* London, 1883.

Severin, Frank T., ed. *Humanistic Viewpoints in Psychology: A Book of Readings.* New York, 1965.

Simon, H. A. "The Architecture of Complexity," *General Systems*, X (1965).

Sinnott, Edmund W. *Cell and Psyche: The Biology of Purpose.* New York, 1961.

Smuts, J. C. *Holism and Evolution.* London, 1926.

Soll, Ivan. *An Introduction to Hegel's Metaphysics.* Chicago, 1969.

Sorokin, P. A. *Contemporary Sociological Theories.* New York, 1928.

Spence, Kenneth W. "Historical and Modern Conceptions of Psychology," *in* E. H. Madden, ed., *The Structure of Scientific Thought.* Boston, 1960.

Spencer, Herbert. *Essays on Education.* London, 1949.

——— *First Principles.* London, 1946.

——— *The Principles of Sociology.* New York, 1895.

Bibliography

——— "The Social Organism," *in* Spencer, *Essays: Scientific, Political, and Speculative*. London, 1863.

Taylor, A. E. *Elements of Metaphysics*. London, 1961.

Teilhard de Chardin, Pierre. *The Phenomenon of Man* (2d ed.). New York, 1965.

Thayer, Frederick. "General System(s) Theory: The Promise That Could Not Be Kept," *Academy of Management Journal*, XV (1972).

Turner, Terence. "Piaget's Structuralism," *American Anthropologist*, LXXV (1973).

Walmsley, D. J. *Systems Theory: A Framework for Human Geographical Enquiry*. Canberra, 1972.

Wann, T. W., ed. *Behaviorism and Phenomenology*. Chicago, 1964.

Watkins, J. W. N. "The Alleged Inadequacy of Methodological Individualism," *Journal of Philosophy*, LV (1958).

——— "Historical Explanation in the Social Sciences," *in* Patrick Gardiner, ed., *Theories of History*. New York, 1959.

——— "Ideal Types and Historical Explanation," *in* H. Feigl and M. Brodbeck, eds., *Readings in the Philosophy of Science*. New York, 1953.

Weiss, Paul. "The Living System: Determinism Stratified," *in* Koestler and Smythies, *Beyond Reductionism*.

——— "1 + 1 ≠ 2 (One Plus One Does Not Equal Two)," *in* G. C. Quarton, T. Melnechuk, and F. O. Schmitt, eds., *The Neurosciences: A Study Program*. New York, 1967.

Werner, Heinz. *Comparative Psychology of Mental Development* (rev. ed.). New York, 1957.

Whitehead, A. N. *Process and Reality*. Cambridge, Eng., 1929.

——— *Science and the Modern World*. New York, 1948.

Woodworth, Robert S. *Contemporary Schools of Psychology*. London, 1952.

Index

Index

Haldane, J. S. and R. B., 25–27, 60
Hayek, F. A. von, 43
Hegel, G. W. F., 7–11 *passim*, 111.
  See also Hegelian philosophy
Hegelian philosophy, 1, 9, 80;
  and theory of internal rela-
  tions, 2, 3, 7–12 *passim*, 16–20
  passim, 49, 61, 110, 123; and
  Bertrand Russell, 11; and John
  Dewey, 49–50, 53, 109; and
  GST, 49, 55, 60–61, 65; and
  David Easton, 78. *See also*
  Hegel, G. W. F.; Holism;
  Organicism
Hempel, Carl, 94–96 *passim*, 123
Heterogeneity, *see* Homogeneity
Hierarchical systems, 35, 69–79
  passim. *See also* Holism 3;
  System
Historicism, 40, 104–6
Holism, 1–4, 121–23; and func-
  tionalism, 2, 94–95, 100; metho-
  dological, 37–45 *passim*, 58;
  and structuralism, 84–89; and
  psychology, 113–21. *See also*
  Bertalanffy, Ludwig von;
  Hegelian philosophy; Social
  sciences
—Holism 1, 6–21 *passim*, 26f, 73–
  74, 77, 86, 101, 110, 122–23;
  and Paul Weiss, 30–35; defined, 36; and methodological
  individualism, 38–44, 113;
  and GST, 46, 48, 57. *See*
  also Functionalism; Gestalt
  psychology; Organicism;
  Structuralism
—Holism 2, 79, 121–23; and Paul
  Weiss, 30–36 *passim*; and
  methodological individualism,
  38–44 *passim*; and Arthur
  Koestler, 73–74; and struc-

turalism, 86–87 *passim*. *See*
  also Analytic method; Reduc-
  tionism
—Holism 3, 122–23; and Paul
  Weiss, 30, 35f; defined, 37; and
  methodological individualism,
  38, 44; and Arthur Koestler,
  69–75. *See also* Analytic
  method
Holon, 69–75. *See also* Koestler,
  Arthur; Whole
Homogeneity, 92, 103. *See also*
  Complexity
Huxley, T. H., 102

Individualism, 2, 37–44, 113. *See*
  also Analytic method; Mech-
  anism; Society
Information theory, 64
Interaction, 51–53, 59, 60ff, 77.
  See also Dewey, John
Interactionism, doctrine of
  universal, 117
Internal relations, theory of, *see*
  Hegelian philosophy
Interrelation, 13, 17, 19, 26, 58,
  62, 78–79, 119; principle of,
  108–9, 110. *See also*
  Continuity

James, William, 53–54, 57f, 62,
  97, 98, 111

Kallen, Horace, 89, 100
Kinship, 84–88 *passim*. *See also*
  Structuralism; Tribe
Knowledge, 50; of whole vs.
  parts, 11, 13, 29, 33–34, 57–58.
  See also Analytic method;
  Hegelian philosophy
Koestler, Arthur, 68–75
Koffka, Kurt, 114, 119

Index

Index

Relations, 7–12, 50, 82–88, 94.
    See also Interrelation
Repression, 102–3
Russell, Bertrand, 11, 29, 46
Ryan, Alan, 94–95, 100

Science, 1, 12, 19, 36, 65–66, 104ff,
    115–16, 121, 123. *See also*
    Biology; Laws; Social sciences
Self-action, level of, 51
Self-regulation, 84, 94–95, 100
Shaw, George Bernard, 25
Smuts, Jan Christian, 29
Social sciences, 1, 66, 106, 122–23.
    See also Anthropology; Psy-
    chology; Sociology
Societal facts, 40–42 *passim*
Societal laws, 41
Society, 80, 91–92, 95–97 *passim*,
    101–6 *passim*. *See also* Collec-
    tivism; Organicism; Sociology;
    Spencer, Herbert; Tribe
Sociology, 2, 37, 95–99 *passim*,
    104, 111–12. *See also* Durk-
    heim, Emile; Individualism;
    Merton, Robert K.; Society;
    Spencer, Herbert
Spencer, Herbert, 80, 89–97
    passim, 103f
Structuralism, 2, 81–89, 102;
    definitions, 81f, 88, 105
Structure, 80–89 *passim*
Sum of the parts, 6, 14f, 33, 39,
    74, 77. *See also* Holism 1;
    Parts; Whole
Synchronic, 88–89, 103–5, 106–11,
    passim
System, 16, 35, 45–54 *passim*, 60–
    64 *passim*, 84–85, 117–18;
    theory, 2, 9, 55–74 *passim*, 75–
    79, 100; analysis, 75–79, 103;

and structuralism, 80, 84–88
    passim; and functionalism, 95,
    100–106 *passim*. *See also* GST;
    Holism 1; Organicism; Or-
    ganism; Tribe

Taylor, A. E., 7, 17, 109
Teleology, 37, 44–45, 67, 93–95,
    100, 102. *See also* Causation
Thorndike, E. L., 115
Topology, 64
Transaction, 51–52, 56–57. *See
    also* Dewey, John
Transformation, 84. *See also*
    Structuralism
Transformational method, 83.
    See also Structuralism
Tribe, 92–93, 95–97 *passim*
Troubetzkoy, N., 83

Virchow, Rudolf, 24
Vitalism, 24–25. *See also*
    Mechanism

Watkins, J. W. N., 38–44 *passim*
Weiss, Paul, 30–36, 38, 42, 68
Wertheimer, Max, 114, 117, 119
Whitehead, A. N., 29
Whole, 1–20 *passim*, 28–29, 47–
    49, 110, 123; vs. parts, 1–20
    passim, 26–29, 53–55, 69–70, 74,
    100–101, 116, 120, 122; and
    structuralism, 84–88; and
    Gestalt psychology, 114,
    117–18. *See also* Holon; Or-
    ganicism; Organism; Parts;
    Society; System
Wholeness, concept of, 1, 34
Wittgenstein, Ludwig, 10–11
Woodger, J. M., 29
Woodworth, Robert, 120

[149]